The Family Doctor

A PHOTOGRAPHIC ESSAY FROM THE MAYFLOWER TO MANAGED CARE

COMPLIMENTS OF BOEHRINGER INGELHEIM PHARMACEUTICALS, INC.

The Family Doctor

A PHOTOGRAPHIC ESSAY FROM THE MAYFLOWER TO MANAGED CARE

with commentary by J. Lynne Dodson

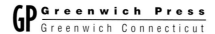

GP **Greenwich Press**
Greenwich Connecticut

Dedication

We dedicate this book and everything it represents to the memory of our friend, Robert Barrett.

Greenwich Press
Greenwich Office Park #6
Greenwich, CT 06830

ISBN: 1-57013-053-1

Group Publisher: Corey Kupersmith, RPh
Publisher: Lynne Kudzy
Editorial Director: Lois Gandt
Art Director: Jill Ruscoll
Designer: Jody Gross

Cover photo: Library of Congress

Every effort has been made to ensure the medical and historical accuracy of this book.
The author regrets any errors, either of fact or omission.

Printed in Hong Kong

Acknowledgments

Grateful acknowledgment is made to many individuals for sharing their expertise and time
and for granting permission to reproduce material from their collections and institutions.
In particular, the following professionals provided invaluable assistance: Karen Anderson,
Michigan Academy of Family Physicians; Alison Barnsley, California Academy of Family Physicians;
Cathy Dyer, Tennessee Academy of Family Physicians; Dr. Karen Gilson; Dr. Henry Gloetzner; Sr. Joan
Marie Hoyt, St. Vincent's Medical Center; John Lovett, University of Oklahoma Library; and Bill Rice,
photography researcher.

About the Photographers

For most of the photographs, tracing the identities of the photographers is impossible. Prints have been
copied and widely distributed, muddying the waters. Most were taken without thought for the historical
perspective they might someday provide. We nevertheless pay tribute to their skill, ingenuity, and
(in some cases) bravado in recording these images for future generations.

Introduction

In one form or another, in all peoples and cultures, some equivalent of the family doctor has been an integral part of the process of healing. The perspective you are about to embark on begins in the 1600s in the Americas with minister-physicians, who were probably the ones best equipped to handle their patients' physical hardships, pestilence-like diseases, and nutritional inadequacies with prayers, kindness, and common sense. Little else was available.

Through the 1700s, university education advanced the practice of medicine, but the overwhelming assaults of disorders such as yellow fever taxed the tools of even the educated clinician. As this book describes, physicians were essential in the advancement of personal and public health during the Revolutionary War by providing advice on personal hygiene, such as an insistence on placing privies a sufficient distance from drinking water to avoid contamination. At a time when 85 percent of military deaths were due to disease, not wounds, an intensive investment of energy was directed toward the development of medications to treat these illnesses.

By the mid-1800s, a flourishing population was supporting the graduation of up to 1000 physicians per year from medical schools, essentially all generalists, who would commonly supplement their otherwise meager medical practice income by such things as farm work.

The introduction of effective anesthesia and beginnings of antisepsis by the 1870s paved the way for increasing frequency of successful surgery, still performed by generalists except in major cities. Most physicians were male, with the first medical degree awarded to a woman in 1849 in New York State.

By the turn of the century, the discovery of x-ray had opened another avenue of medical investigation. As cities developed, so did urban medical centers, which attracted patients by offering sophisticated techniques like x-ray, the comfort of painless surgical procedures thanks to the then well-established techniques of anesthesia, and decreased levels of infection due to appropriate application of antisepsis techniques, all of which promised much more favorable outcomes. Practice styles and economics of family physicians in rural and frontier areas were becoming quite different from those practicing in well-to-do urban areas.

By the early and mid-1900s, a dizzying array of specialty skills were appropriately encouraging development of multiple subspecialties. The capacity to prevent many of the major communicable diseases, treat many of the other infectious diseases, and avoid problems of malnutrition gave the family physician plenty to do.

Development of the family physician role since the 1950s has been substantially affected by an overall abundance of health care providers. Allocation of resources has required clearly defined roles that are in a state of rapid evolution. Studies of the efficacy of family physicians in both cost and patient satisfaction, when compared with other providers, solidifies their position as entry-level providers. Family doctors' effective resource utilization in times of increasingly selective availability has placed them in leadership positions in the medical community hierarchy. Family physicians continue to expand the types of procedures contained within the definition of our specialty, and the end is nowhere in sight.

Looking back after practicing medicine for 23 years now, much has evolved in medicine since the days when my own family doctor came to the house to administer penicillin shots for a respiratory infection, lest the dread rheumatic fever darken our doorway. My parents stood personally over each of us as we swallowed the "sugar cube" containing the first oral polio vaccine and sighed with relief that their children would likely not be victimized.

Sometimes we feel and acknowledge history as it happens. Other times it happens without the politeness of announcing itself. Eventually, we learn the impact of the events we live.

The book you are about to open is a history that reflects the story of not one man or woman, but the collective story of the development of family medicine. Certainly each image contains a past, present, and future that would reveal a remarkable tapestry of events, were we allowed the privilege of full under-standing. However, we must content ourselves with the weave of the tale that is told by capturing just one moment in time. For family physicians reading this book, we hope it speaks to you personally of your own roots and "family of origin" professionally. For other readers, this book offers an overview of the evolution of our profession and clues to what we may further hope for it as our progress continues.

Louis Kuritzky, MD
University of Florida
Gainesville, Florida

Contents

Chapter 1

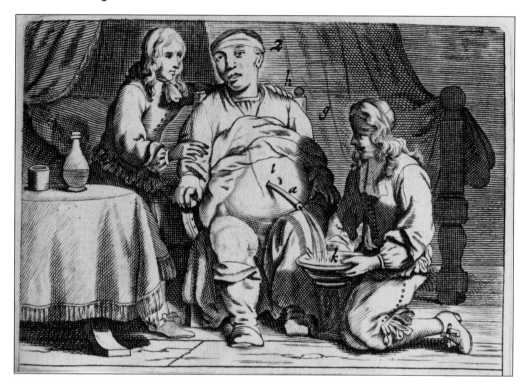

THE FOUNDATIONS OF AMERICAN MEDICINE 1600–1800

To Europe's physicians in the 17th century, colonial America did not appear to be a land of opportunity. These highly educated professionals had little reason to leave their flourishing practices among upper- and middle-class patients to make a hazardous transatlantic voyage to sparsely settled wilderness.

As a result, an eclectic assortment of individuals provided healing services to colonial Americans, a tradition that continued well into the 19th century. Folk practitioners, barber-surgeons, apothecaries, bloodletters, and midwives applied common sense, traditional practices, herbal remedies, and occasionally even "learned medicine" to attempt to cure their fellow settlers.

In the English and Dutch colonies, minister-physicians came to be the predominant health care providers—what one author has termed "the angelic connection." Deacon Dr. Samuel Fuller arrived on the *Mayflower* in 1620; his wife, who arrived three years later, is thought to have been the first midwife in the New England colonies.

However, the presence of trained physicians apparently did not make much difference. In the Virginia colony, physicians arrived with the colonists as early as 1608, assigned by the Virginia Company. Yet of the 9000 people who had arrived by 1625, only about 1200 remained. While a few hundred had returned to England, most had died of the effects of malnutrition, typhoid, malaria, and wounds.

Despite the hardships, by the century's end an estimated 275000 people had settled in the Eastern colonies. The largest city was Boston, with about 7000 inhabitants; New York City had about 5000.

Right: This broadside, published in 1677, was one of the first medical publications in the colonies. As was true of most colonial medical works, it was written "not to inform the Learned Physician...but to give some light to those that have not such advantages." In the early Dutch and English colonies, medical care was commonly provided by ministers, such as the broadside's author, the Rev. Thomas Thacher, and other learned men.

12

A
BRIEF RULE

To guide the Common-People of

NEW-ENGLAND

How to order themselves and theirs in the

Small Pocks, or Measels.

The *small Pox* (whose nature and cure the *Measels* follow) is a disease in the blood, endeavouring to recover a new form and state.

2. This nature attempts----1. By Separation of the impure from the pure, thrusting it out from the Veins to the Flesh.----2. By driving out the impure from the Flesh to the Skin.

3. The first Separation is done in the first four dayes by a Feaverish boyling (Ebullition) of the Blood, laying down the impurities in the Fleshy parts which kindly effected the Feaverish tumult is calmed.

4. The second Separation from the Flesh to the Skin, or *Superficies* is done through the rest of the time of the disease.

5. There are several Errors in ordering these sick ones in both these Operations of Nature which prove very dangerous and commonly deadly either by overmuch hastening Nature beyond its own pace, or in hindering of it from its own vigorous operation.

6. The Separation by Ebullition in the Feaverish heat is oyer heightened by too much Clothes, too hot a room, hot *Cordials*, as *Diascordium*, *Gascons powder* and such like, for hence come *Phrensies*, dangerous excessive sweats, or the flowing of the Pocks into one overspreading fore, vulgarly called the Flox.

7. The same feperation is overmuch hindred by preposterous cooling that Feaverish boyling heat, by *blood letting*, *Glyfters*, *Vomits*, *purges*, or *cooling medicines*. For though these many times haften the coming forth of the *Pox*, yet they take away that supply which should keep them out till they are ripe, wherefore they sink in again to the deadly danger of the sick.

8. If a *Phrensie* happen, or through a *Plethoris* (that is fulness of blood) the Circulation of the blood be hindred, and thereupon the whole mass of blood choaked up, then either let blood, Or fee that their diet, or medicines be not altogether cooling, but let them in no wise be heating, therefore let him lye no otherwise covered in his bed then he was wont in health: His Chamber not made hot with fire if the weather be temperate, let him drink small Beer only warm'd with a Toft, let him sup up thin *water-gruel*, or water-pottage made only of Indian Flour and water, instead of *Oat-meal*: Let him eat *boild Apples*: But I would not advise at this time any medicine besides. By this means that exceffive *Ebullition* (or boyling of his blood) will by degrees abate, and the Symptoms ceafe; If not, but the blood be so inraged that it will admit no delay, then either let blood (if Age will bear it) or elfe give some notably cooling medicine, or refresh him with more free Air.

9. But if the boiling of the blood be weak and dull that there is caufe to fear it is not able to work a Separation, as it's wont to be in such as have been let blood, or are fat, or Flegmatick, or brought low by some other sicknefs or labour of the (*Gonorrhea*) running of the Reins, or fome other Evacuation : In such Cafes, *Cordials* must drive them out, or they must dy.

10. In time of driving out the *Pocks* from the Flesh, here care must be had that the *Puftules* keep out in a right meafure till they have attain'd their end without going in again, for that is deadly.

11. In this time take heed when the *Puftules* appear whilft not yet ripe, leaft by too much heat there arise a new *Ebullition* (or Feaverish boyling) for this troubles the driving out, or brings back the separated parts into the blood, or the Fleshy parts overheated are disabled from a right suppuration or laftly the temper of the blood and tone of the Flesh is so perverted that it cannot overcome and digeft the matter driven out.

12. Yet on the other hand the breaking out muft not be hindred, by expofing the fick unto the cold. The degree of heat muft be such as is natural agrees with the temper of the fleshy parts : That which exceeds or falls short is dangerous : Therefore the reafon of the year, Age of the fick, and their manner of life here require a difcreet and different Confideration, requiring the Counsel of an expert Phyfitian.

13. But if by any error a new *Ebullition* arifeth, the fame art must be ufed to allay it as is before expreft.

14. If the *Puftles* go in and a flux of the belly follows (for elfe there is no such danger) then *Cordials* are to be ufed, yet moderate and not too often for fear of new *Ebullition*.

15. If much fpitting (*Ptyalifmus*) follow, you may hope all will go well, therefore by no means hinder it : Only with warm small Beer let their mouths be washed.

16. When the *Puftles* are dryed and fallen, purge well, especially if it be in *Autumn*.

17. As soon as this disease therefore appears by its figns, let the sick abftein from Flesh and Wine, and open Air, let him ufe small Bear warmed with a Toft for his ordinary drink, and moderately when he defires it. For food ufe *water-gruel*, *water-pottage*, and other things having no manifeft hot quality, eafy of digeftion, boild Apples, and milk fometimes for change, but the coldnefs taken off. Let the ufe of his bed be according to the feafon of the year, and the multitude of the *Pocks*, or as found perfons

are wont: In Summer let him rife according to cuftome, yet fo as to be defended both from heat and cold in Excefs, the diseafe will be the fooner over and lefs troublefome, for being kept in bed nourifheth the Feaverish heat and makes the Pocks break out with a painful inflamation.

19. In a colder feafon, and breaking forth of a multitude of *Puftules*, forcing the fick to keep his bed, let him be covered according to his cuftome in health, a moderate fire in the winter being kindled in his Chamber, morning and Evening : neither need he keep his Arms alwayes in bed, or ly ftill in the fame place, for fear leaft he should fweat which is very dangerous efpecially to youth.

20. Before the fourth day ufe no medicines to drive out, nor be too ftrict with the fick; for by how much the more gently the *Puftules* do grow, by fo much the fuller and perfecter will the Separation be.

21. On the fourth day a gentle *Cordial* may help once given.

22. From that time a small draught of warm milk (not hot) a little dy'd with *Saffron* may be given morning and evening till the *Puftules* are come to their due greatnefs and ripenefs.

23. When the *Puftules* begin to dry and cruft, leaft the rotten vapours ftrike inward, which fometimes caufeth fudden death; Take morning and evening some temperate *Cordial* as four or five fpoonfuls of *Malago wine* tinged with a little *Saffron*.

24. When the *Puftules* are dryd and fallen off, purge once and again, especially in the *Autumn Pocks*.

25. Beware of anointing with *Oils*, *Fatts*, *Ointments*, and such defenfives, for keeping the corrupted matter in the *Puftules* from drying up, by the moisture they fret deeper into the Flesh, and fo make the more deep Scarrs.

26. The young and lively men that are brought to a plentiful fweat in this ficknefs, about the eighth day the fweat ftops of it self, by no means afterwards to be drawn out again; the fick thereupon feels moft troublefome difreft and anguish, and then makes abundance of water and fo dyes.

Few young men and ftrong thus handled efcape, except they fall into abundance of fpitting or plentiful bleeding at the nofe.

27. Signs difcovering the Affault at firft are beating pain in the head, Forehead, and temples, pain in the back, great fleepinefs, gliftring of the eyes, fhining glimmerings feem before them, itching of them alfo, with tears flowing of themfelves, itching of the Nofe, short breath, dry Cough, oft neezing, hoarfenefs, heat, rednefs, and fenfe of pricking over the whole body, terrors in the fleep, forrow and reftlefnefs, beating of the heart, *Urine* fometimes in health, fometime filthy from great *Ebullition*, and all this or many of thefe with a Feaverish diftemper.

28. Signs warning of the probable Event. If they break forth eafily, quickly, and foon come to ripening; if the Symptoms be gentle, the Feaver mild, and after the breaking forth it abates If the voice be free, and breathing eafie, efpecially if the Pox be red white, diftinct, foft few, round, sharp top'd, only without and not in the inward parts; if there be large bleeding at the nofe. Thefe figns are hopeful.

29. But such figns are doubtful, when they difficultly appear, when they fink in again, when they are black, blewish, green, hard, all in one, if the Feaver abate not with their breaking forth, if there be Swooning, difficulty of breathing, great thirft, quinfey, great unquietnefs, and it is very dangerous, if there be ioyn'd with it fome other malignant Feaver, called by fome the peftilential Pox: the *Spotted Feaver* is oft joyned with it.

30. Deadly Signs if the *Flux* of the *Belly* happen, when they are broke forth, if the Urine be bloody, or black, or the *Ordure* of that Colour, Or if pure blood be caft out by the Belly or Gumms: Thefe Signs are for the moft part deadly.

Thefe things have I written Candid Reader, *not to inform the* Learned Phyfitian *that hath much more caufe to underftand what pertains to this disease than I, but to give fome light to thofe that have not such advantages, leaving the difficulty of this difeafe to the* Phyfitians Art, wifdome, and Faithfulnefs *: for the right managing of them in the whole Courfe of the disease tends both to the Patients fafety, and the* Phyfitians *defired Succefs in his Adminiftrations: For in vain is the* Phyfitians Art imployed, *if they are not under a* Regular Regiment. *I am, though no* Phyfitian, *yet a well wisher to the sick: And therefore intreating the* Lord *to turn our hearts, and ftay his hand, I am*

21. 11. 167⅞.

A Friend, Reader to thy
Welfare,

Thomas Thacher.

BOSTON, Printed and fold by *John Foster*. 1677.

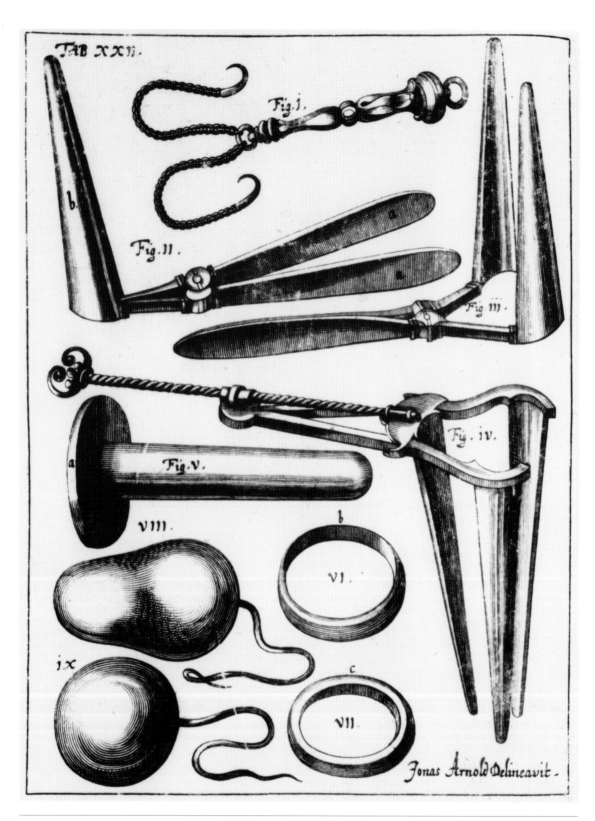

This illustration of obstetrical instruments is from Joannis Scultetus' Armamentarium Chirurgicum, *1665 edition. Midwives landed with the first women settlers and handled almost all obstetrical cases. Childbirth was a significant cause of death for colonial women, with or without a physician in attendance.*

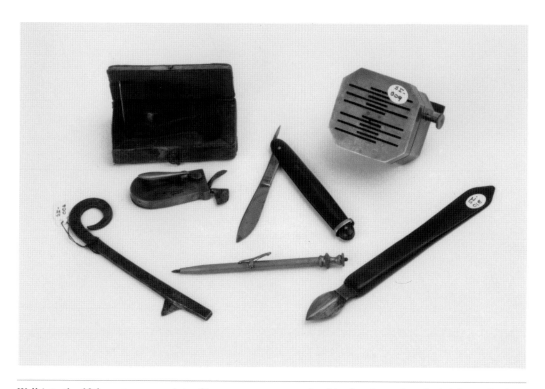

Well into the 19th century, a variety of instruments were used to bleed patients. In colonial days a barber-surgeon, bloodletter, or physician might remove as much as a quart of blood in a 48-hour period. The procedure was thought to reduce excitability in the blood, thereby lowering fevers.

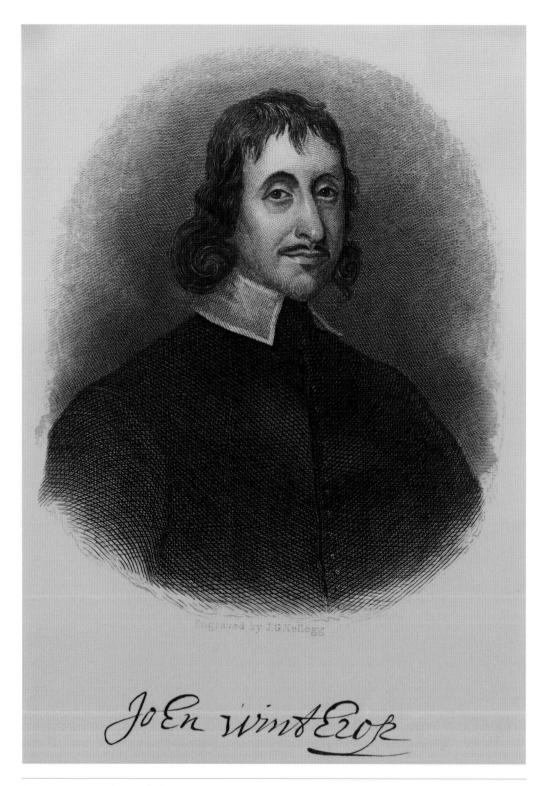

Engraved by J.G.Kellogg

Given a scarcity of trained physicians, any well-read citizen might be called on to care for the sick. Connecticut's governor John Winthrop, Jr., was well known as a healer; he also carried out experiments in alchemy and was elected to membership in the Royal Society of London.

The 18th century saw no real developments in general medical therapy in either Europe or the colonies, except for growing acceptance of inoculation against smallpox in America. Physicians continued to bleed, blister, purge, and sweat their patients.

That is not to say, however, that other aspects of colonial medicine were static. By the time of the Revolutionary War, America had about 3500 practicing physicians, 400 of whom had received university degrees. The country also had its first general hospital, the Pennsylvania Hospital, and its own medical school, the Philadelphia Medical College. Three more medical schools would be founded by the end of the century.

An American medical publishing establishment developed, at first primarily printing colonial editions of popular European works. *Every Man His Own Doctor: Or, the Poor Planter's Physician* by Virginian John Tennent and William Buchan's *Domestic Medicine* underwent numerous reprints. The first publication on surgery to be written and printed in the colonies was a treatise on the treatment of wounds and fractures by John Jones in 1775. Other works included a clinical account of a scarlet fever outbreak in Boston in 1735 by Dr. William Douglass and an essay by Cadwallader Colden on the 1741 epidemic of yellow fever in New York City.

The Revolutionary War was a major stimulus to the development of medicine in the colonies. America's first pharmacopoeia was published by Physician-General Dr. William Brown for use by the military hospital staff. During the war, Congress established the position of Apothecary-General, equal in rank and pay to the Surgeon-General, and added apothecaries to the staff of the military hospital. This would help establish the specialty in its own right. Preventive medicine also received a boost. With six of seven military deaths caused by disease, not injuries, interest became focused on hygiene and camp sanitation. Even rank-and-file soldiers came to recognize the value of published advice by Physician-General Dr. Benjamin Rush on the importance of bathing regularly, airing tents, and siting privies on the outskirts of camps.

Despite repeated epidemics, by the first census of 1790, the new American nation had 3.9 million inhabitants.

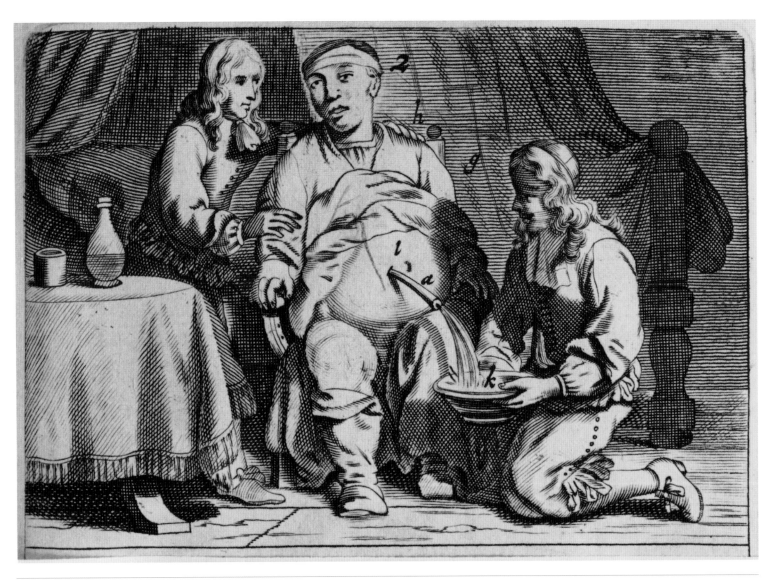

Treatment of a patient with dropsy involved tapping the abdomen to reduce the fluid accumulation. This illustration appeared in the 1741 edition of Scultetus' Armamentarium Chirurgicum.

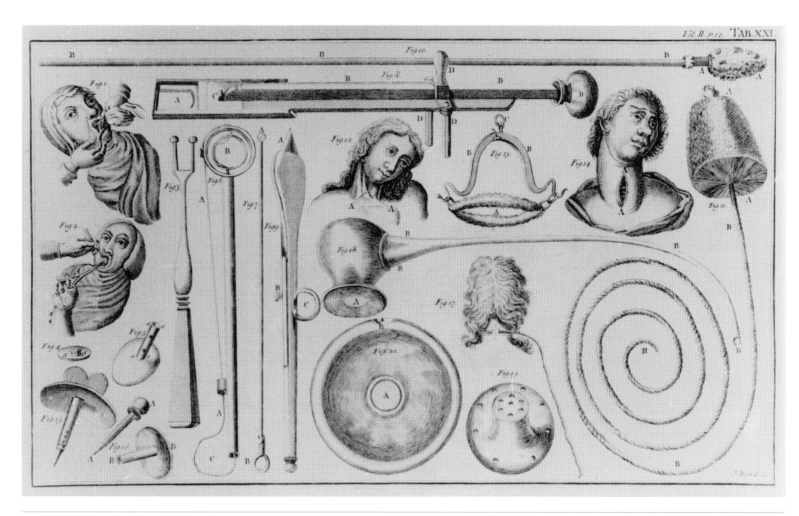

At the time of the Revolutionary War, most of the practicing physicians in the colonies had learned their profession by apprenticing for three to six years with an experienced physician or by reading books, such as this highly influential illustrated text, A General System of Surgery, *by Lorenz Heister.*

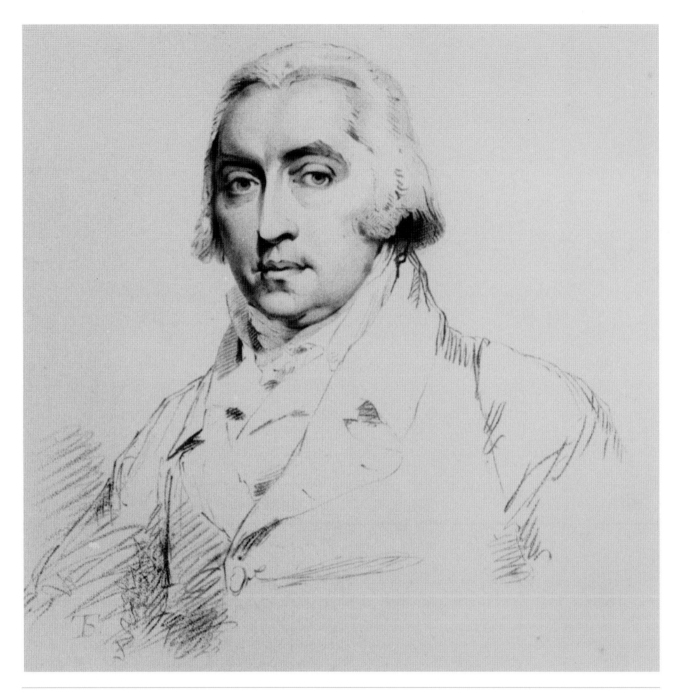

Above: Dr. Philip Syng Physick received his medical degree from Edinburgh University in 1792 and quickly established himself as a skilled surgeon in the colonies. At that time, even prominent surgeons had thriving general practices. Physick, for example, developed the technique of bleeding a patient to unconsciousness in order to replace dislocated joints manually.

Right: Without anesthesia or antiseptics, it is not surprising that few patients submitted to major surgery willingly. Amputations were the most common major procedure, although by the end of the 18th century, physicians were removing cataracts and tonsils, correcting harelip, and excising tumors. This illustration is from Benjamin Bell's A System of Surgery, *the first American edition of which was published in 1791.*

PLATE LXXXI

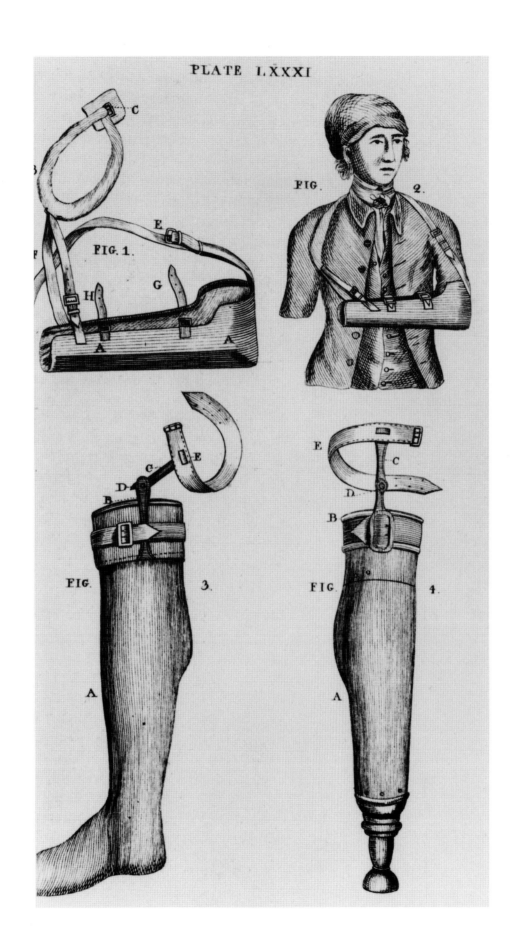

Chapter 2

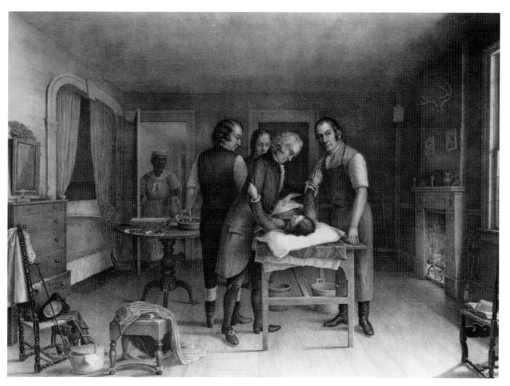

THE VERSATILE
AMERICAN PHYSICIAN
1801–1865

The 19th century would bring significant changes to America and to its medical profession. In the ten years since the first census (1790), the population had increased by 35%. Western migration would eventually take thousands, including some physicians and apothecaries, into the Louisiana, Northwest, and Western territories.

Medicine would undergo its own growth spurt. In the 35 years from 1765 to 1800, American medical schools graduated 250 physicians. In the single decade of the 1850s, almost 18 000 physicians were graduated, nearly all of them general practitioners. While a few of the best qualified would support themselves entirely by caring for their well-to-do city-dwelling patients, most physicians throughout the century would have to supplement their medical income with earnings from a farm or other business.

Perhaps the most significant medical development of the period would be the introduction of anesthesia in surgery. This would allow surgeons to carry out major procedures without hurrying and to explore the internal organs and processes. Within 20 years, Lister would show the effectiveness of antisepsis and establish the validity of work by Pasteur and Koch on the bacteria theory of infection, and surgery would never be the same. While rural and frontier physicians would continue to perform surgery, surgical specialization would soon be a fact of life for American physicians.

Right: As the population moved rapidly westward out of the coastal urban centers, entrepreneurs saw opportunities to prosper from the urgent need for frontier doctors. With no legal regulations or organized standards in effect, proprietary medical schools offered a medical diploma with as few as 14 weeks of training. As many as 400 medical schools operated in the United States in the 19th century, graduating nearly 18 000 students in the 1850s. The Kansas Medical College of Topeka eventually affiliated with an established university and became the Washburn College School of Medicine.

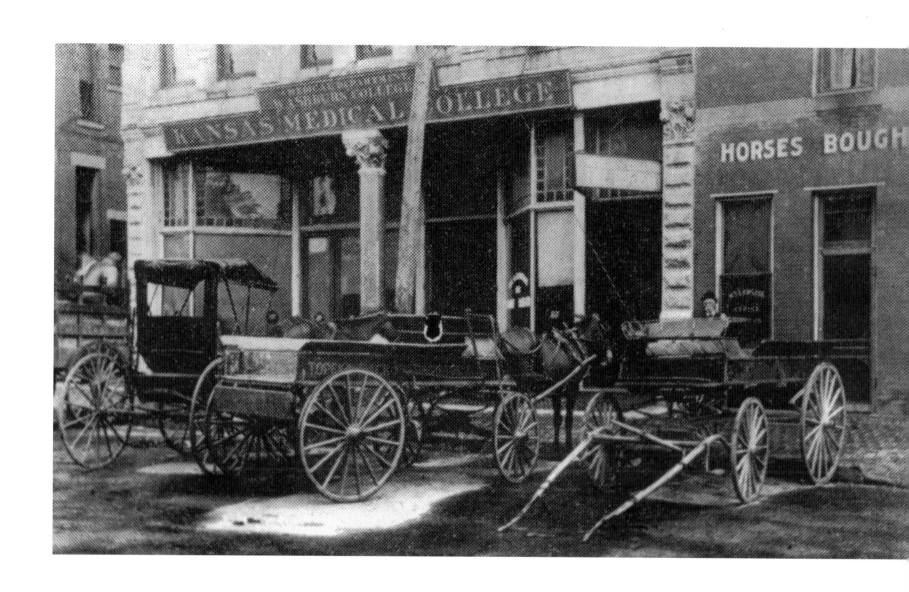

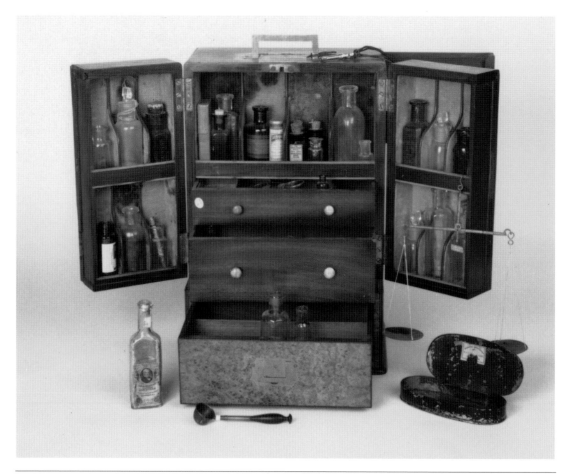

As cities grew, physicians and apothecaries or pharmacists tended to work within their respective fields. However, the country physician was often called on to make the compounds he prescribed, as this portable medicine cabinet, made in 1832, indicates. In the rear is a hidden compartment for narcotics. Laudanum, a tincture of opium, was especially popular for relief of pain and inflammation. By the 1890s, Americans were using 500 000 pounds of crude opium annually in a variety of forms.

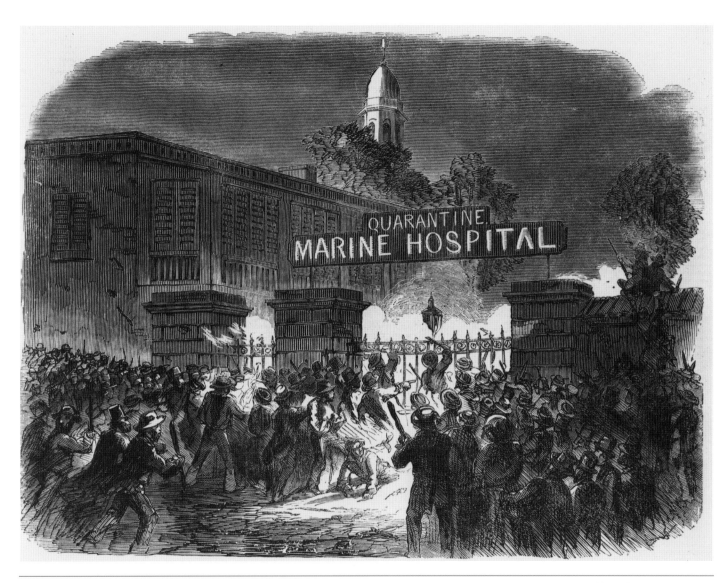

Epidemics of smallpox, yellow fever, and cholera wreaked havoc in many populous areas during the 19th century, especially in the port cities. Smallpox, which had afflicted 75% of the population of Charleston, South Carolina, during a 1760 epidemic, declined in frequency as vaccination became common early in the 19th century. Yellow fever became less of a threat in New England during the century's first decade, but ravaged the South throughout most of the remaining 90 years. This illustration, from the September 11, 1858, Harper's Weekly, *depicts an attack by local citizens on the quarantine hospital, which they believed was "breeding pestilence" and harming the city.*

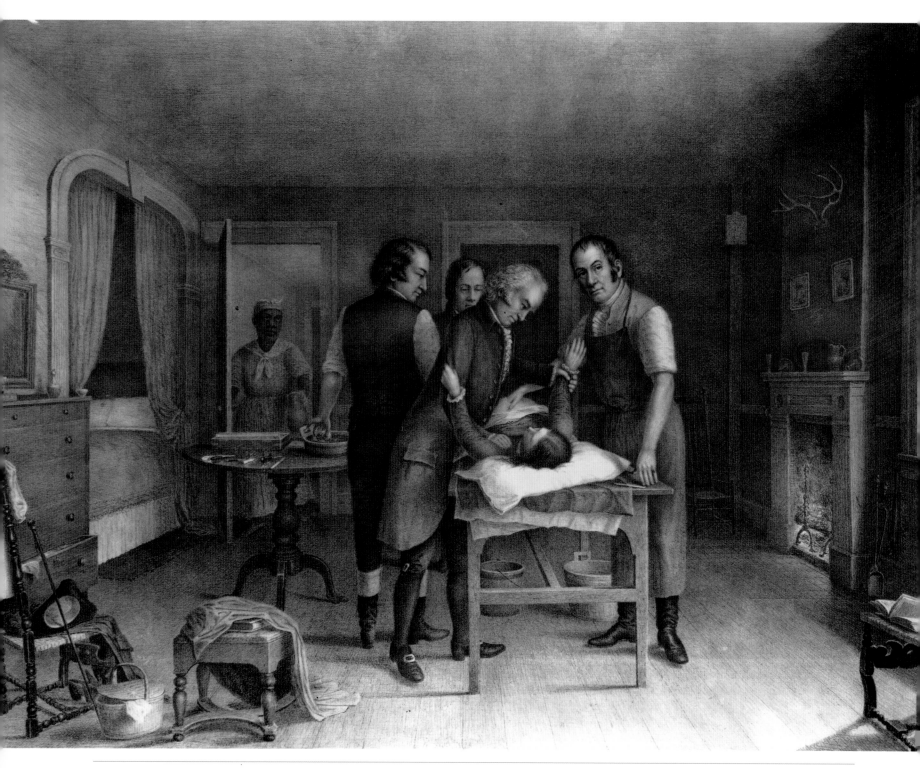

In December 1809, Dr. Ephraim McDowell of Danvillé, Kentucky, made medical history by successfully removing a 20-pound ovarian cyst from Jane Crawford, who had traveled 60 miles on horseback to undergo the procedure in McDowell's home. Anesthesia was not yet available, although opium was often used to dull pain. Mrs. Crawford repeated the Psalms throughout the surgery and 25 days later rode back to her own home, living for another 31 years.

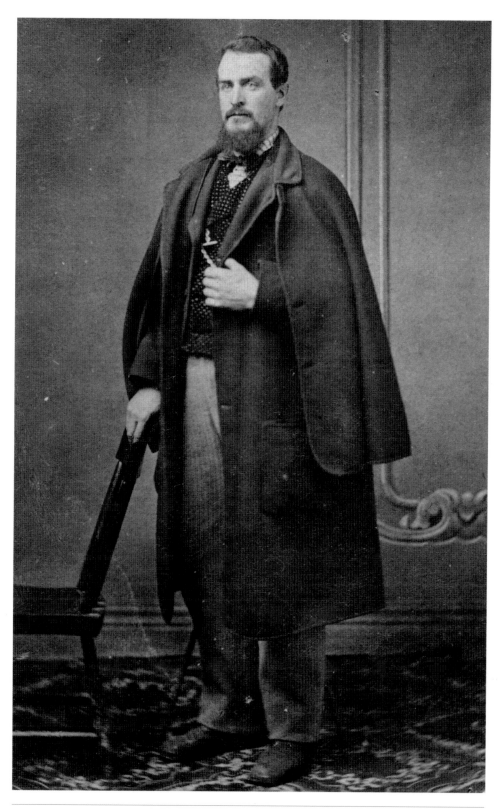

Dr. L. Rodney Pococke was the first physician known to have set up practice in Helena, Montana. However, just two years later in 1865, his was the first recorded death in Helena—of consumption.

Chapter 3

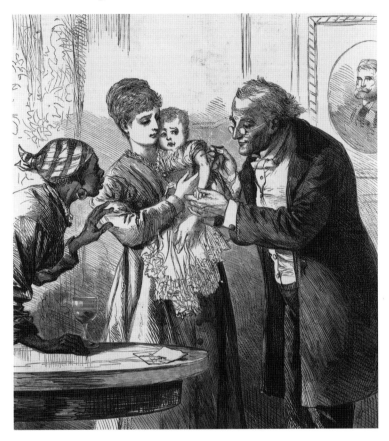

DECADES OF CHANGE
1866-1900

Although many physicians and their patients were probably not aware of it, the medical profession at the end of the 19th century was considerably different from what it had been at the beginning of that century.

One significant factor was the changes that were being made in medical education. In 1893 Johns Hopkins University Medical School opened, a noteworthy event for several reasons:

- Applicants had to have a bachelor's degree and a knowledge of French and German.
- No applicant could be refused admission because of gender.
- Students were required to undergo a clinical rotation at a hospital that was permanently staffed by Johns Hopkins faculty.
- The school's endowment included a research laboratory, helping to integrate clinical and research medicine.

Other medical schools and professional organizations were also working to strengthen medical education. The University of Pennsylvania implemented entrance examinations for medical school admission in 1881. In 1894, after an earlier attempt failed, the National Association of Medical Colleges voted to increase the course of study to four years. And in 1900 the American Medical Association delegates voted to refuse membership to anyone with less than four years of training.

Medical technology would contribute to the changing profession as well. Stethoscopes, thermometers, and x-ray devices helped physicians better understand and describe internal processes. Unfortunately, however, improvements in diagnosis were not accompanied by advances in treatment.

The country had changed, too. At the first census in 1790, only 4% of Americans lived in cities; at the 1900 census, nearly 40% of the 76 million Americans lived in urban areas—many in slums with unhealthy conditions.

Right: The country doctor needed "an extra measure of physical stamina, ingenuity approaching genius, and a philosophy of life to bear up under professional strains and personal adversity," wrote one expert on frontier medicine. These practitioners were usually viewed by their patients as a symbol of hope during bleak times.

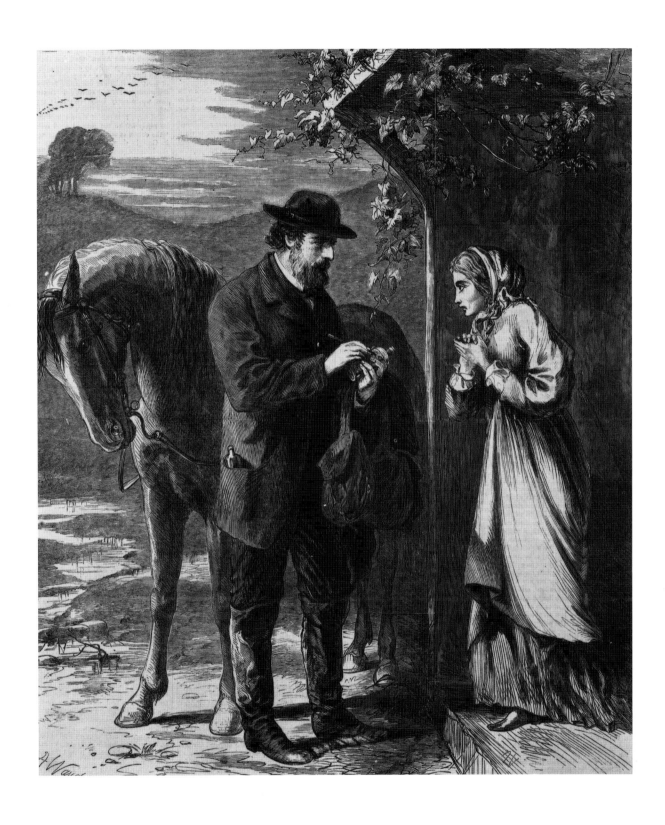

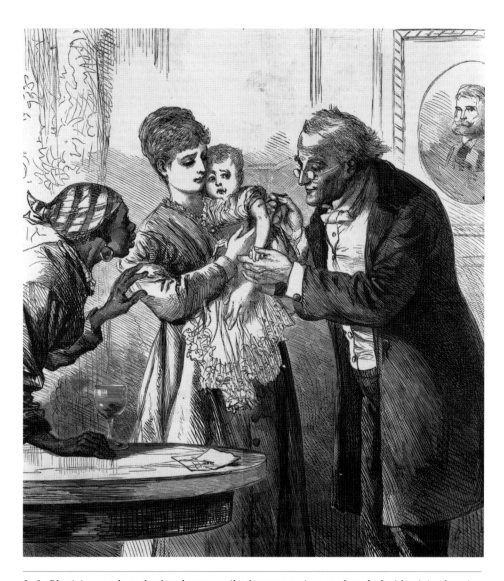

Left: Physicians on horseback rode many miles between patients and worked with minimal equipment and few drugs. They might be called on to perform surgery under a tree, on a wagon bed, or on a kitchen table.

Above: In urban areas, young physicians usually sought a family practice among the well-to-do. In such circumstances, a physician could make a comfortable living and enjoy a level of social status, caring for the families and their servants in their homes. However, as too many physicians had clustered in the cities, most had to settle for much less.

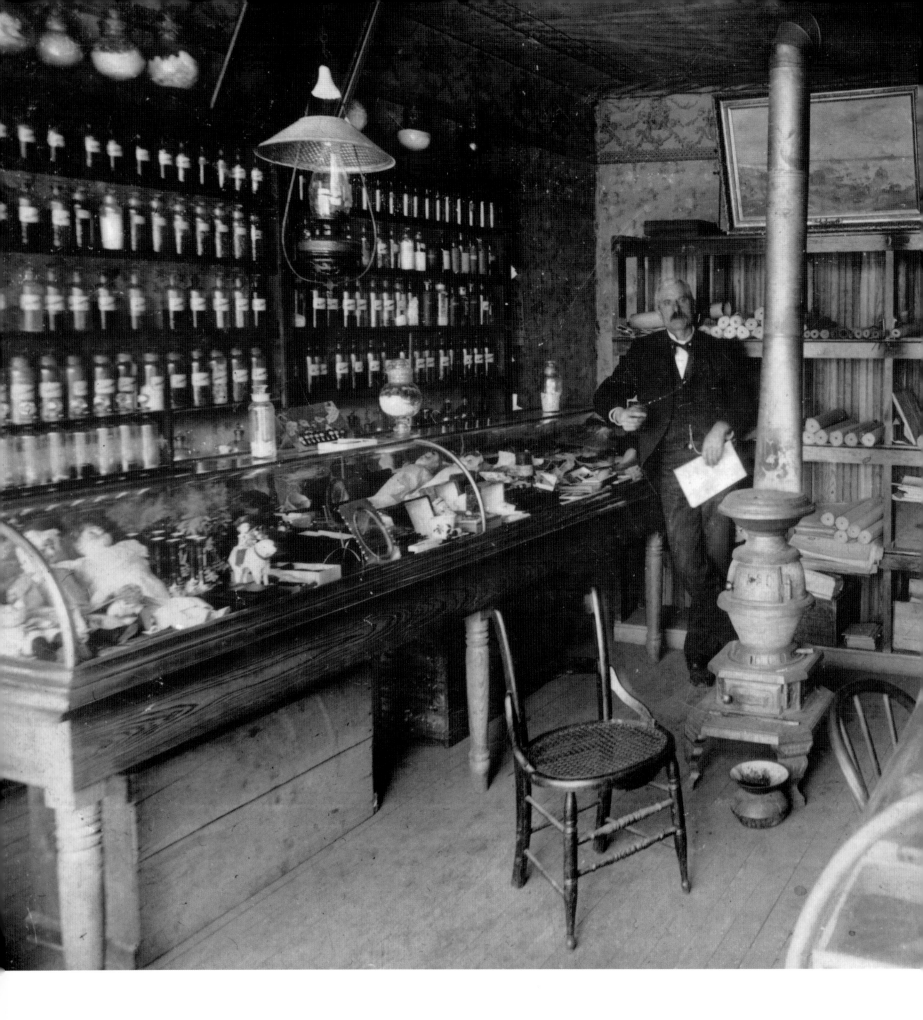

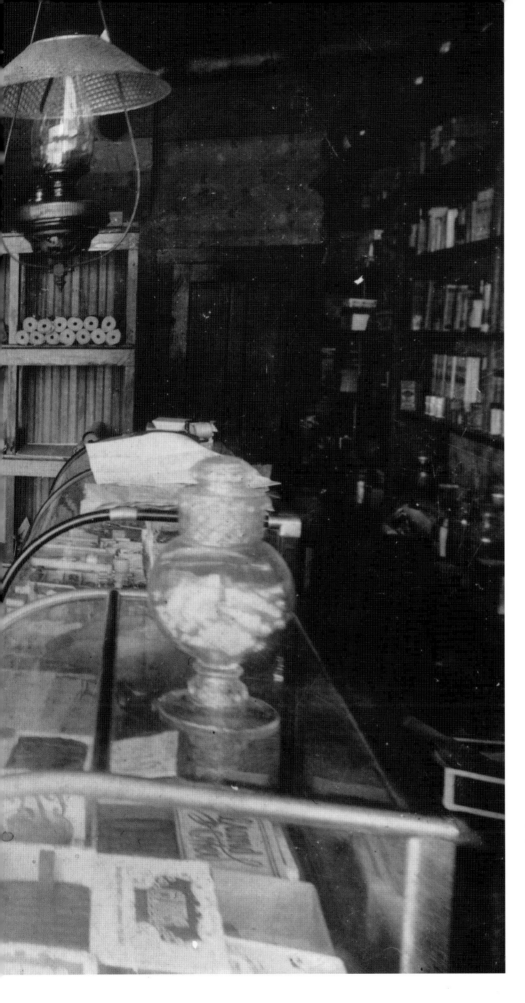

Most pioneer physicians had to supplement their practice income. Farming, mining, and various businesses were among the common means of support. Dr. James Raizon of Trinidad, Colorado, like many other physicians, operated his own drugstore. In addition to the drugs he compounded, the store offered toys, candy, wallpaper, tobacco, and numerous sundry items. Eventually, the soda fountain would replace a chair and spitoon as a place for locals to gather.

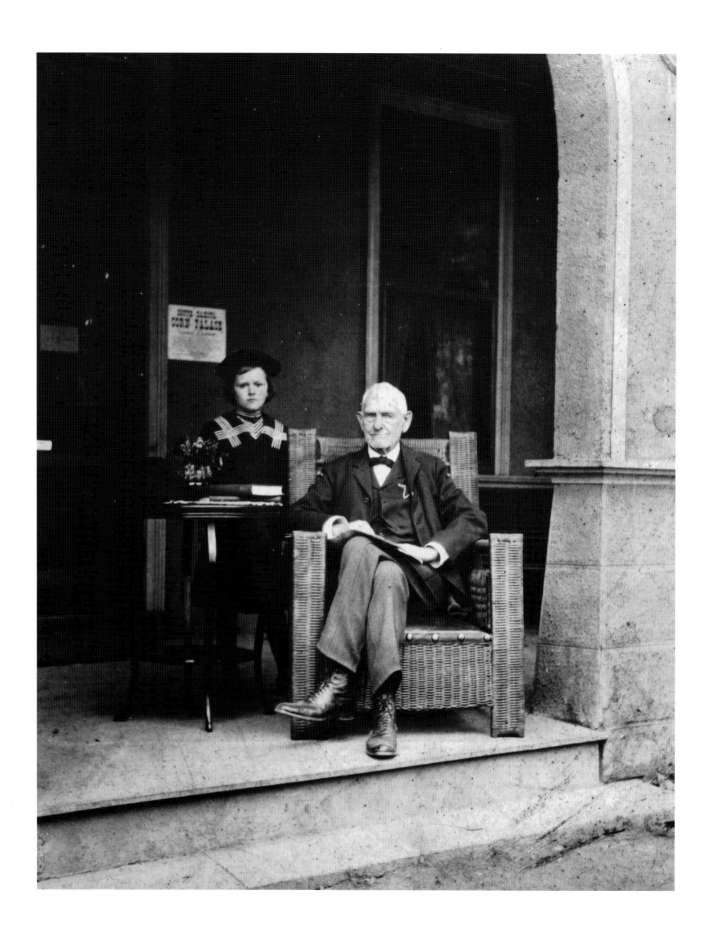

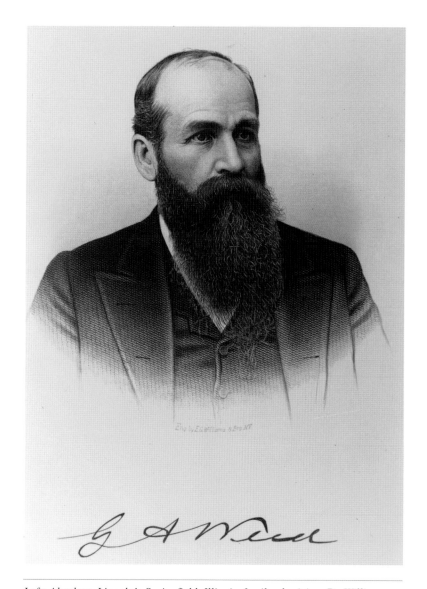

Left: Abraham Lincoln's Springfield, Illinois, family physician, Dr. William Jayne, was appointed by President Lincoln as governor of the Dakota Territory. Later he would be elected a territorial delegate to Congress before returning to Springfield.

Above: Frontier physicians were often among the most educated citizens in their communities and became politically and socially active. Dr. Gideon Weed was twice elected mayor of Seattle, Washington, and established a hospital in the city in 1874. He became wealthy through various real estate dealings.

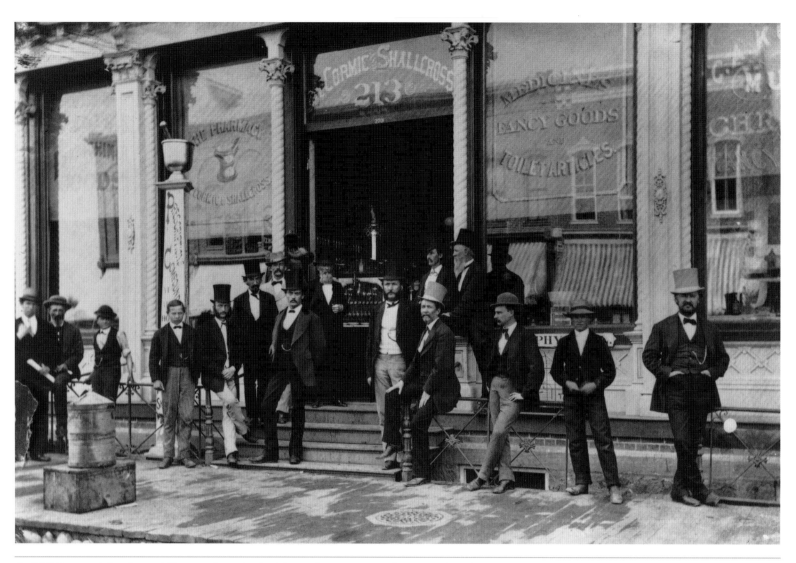

By 1873 Denver, Colorado, could boast at least six physicians, who were among this group of gentlemen to pose in front of the McCormic and Shallcross Drugstore.

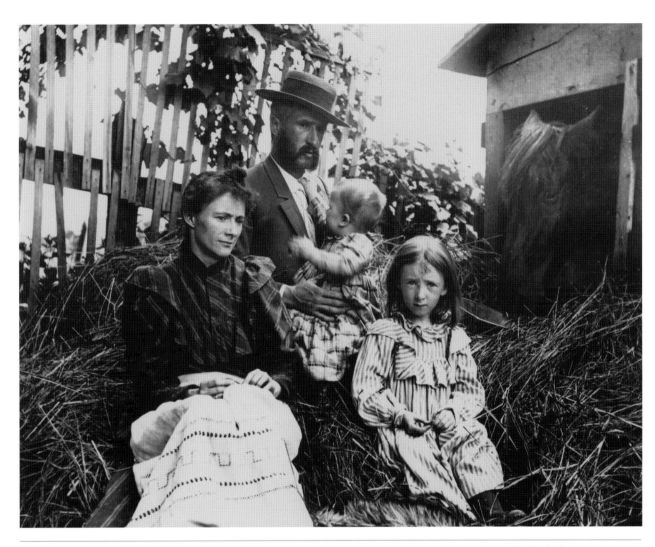

The pivotal role that horses played in the practice of frontier medicine is indicated by the frequency with which their names are noted in doctors' reminiscences. A good horse could be counted on to guide the doctor home through blizzards or a much-needed nap. Wisconsin doctor Edward Bass and his family posed with his valued steed, "Dick."

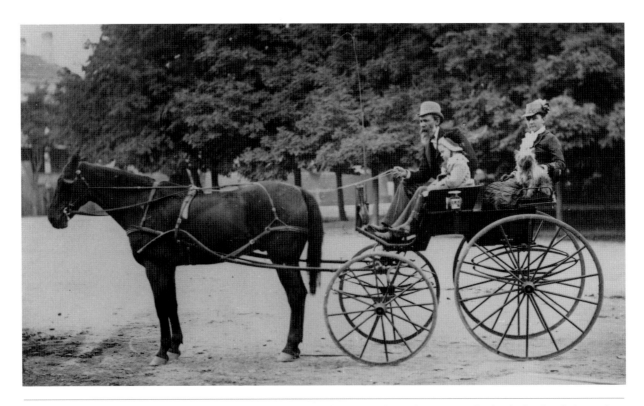

Dr. John F. Hamilton and his family are shown in his four-wheel carriage, favored over two-wheel vehicles for their comfort and tendency to remain upright when riding over rocks. Buggies could, of course, carry more equipment than a horse and so were the preferred means of transport when travel was over roads or flat land to patients.

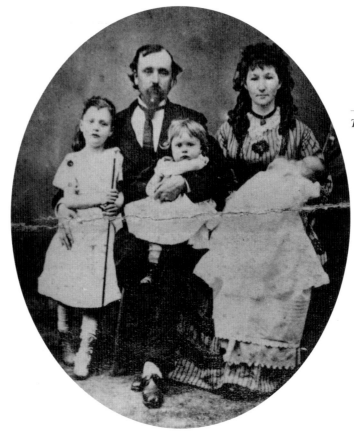

The Dakotas were still a territory in 1876 when Dr. Benjamin Slaughter posed with his wife, Linda, and their daughters, Roselind, Jessamine, and Linnie Lee. On average, the girls could expect to live into their early or mid forties.

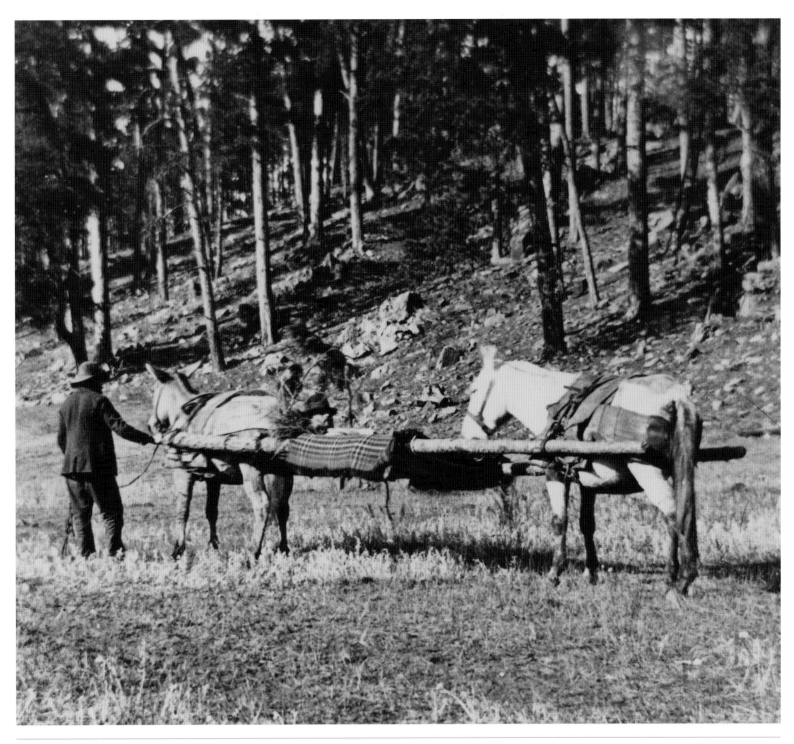

Frontier physicians, like the people they cared for, learned to make do with what was at hand. Adaptability under unusual circumstances and inventive genius were essential to the survival of both doctor and patient. Here a man, reportedly wounded at the battle of Slim Buttes, is carried on a stretcher made from small tree trunks and blankets, with dried grass for a pillow and a pine branch to provide shade.

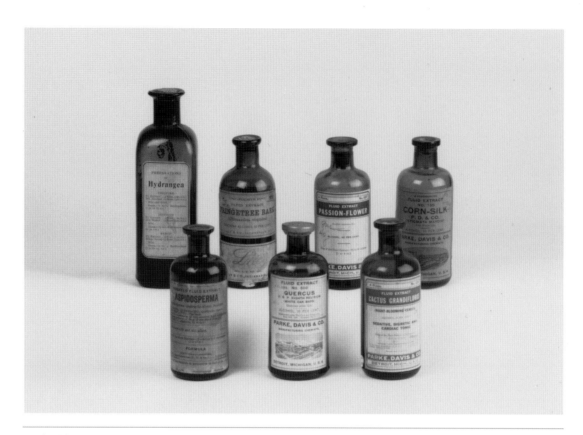

Medical botany had arrived with the first practitioners to the colonies. In 1798 Benjamin Smith Barton issued a pioneer compilation of American plant drugs. However, by the late 19th century botanicals were largely abandoned by "regular" physicians. These extracts and compounds, prescribed as diuretics, antispasmodics, and stimulants, would be increasingly replaced by metallic substances and compounds.

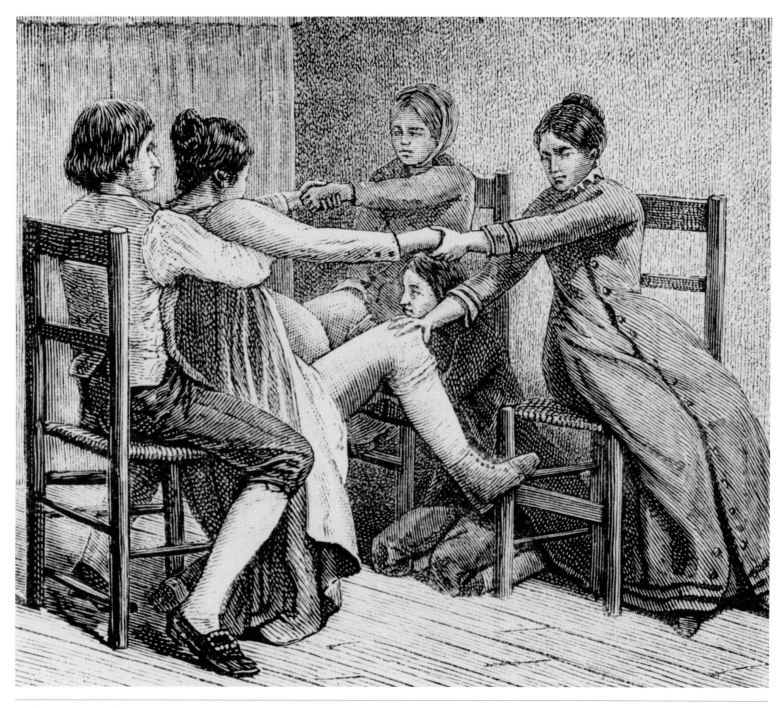

In the cities the developing specialty of obstetrics would push midwives away from the birth scene for upper- and middle-class women by the 1830s. Frontier conditions, however, often called for assistance from any practitioner within traveling distance. With her husband acting as a "birthing chair," this pioneer woman is assisted by both a physician and midwives in this 1887 engraving.

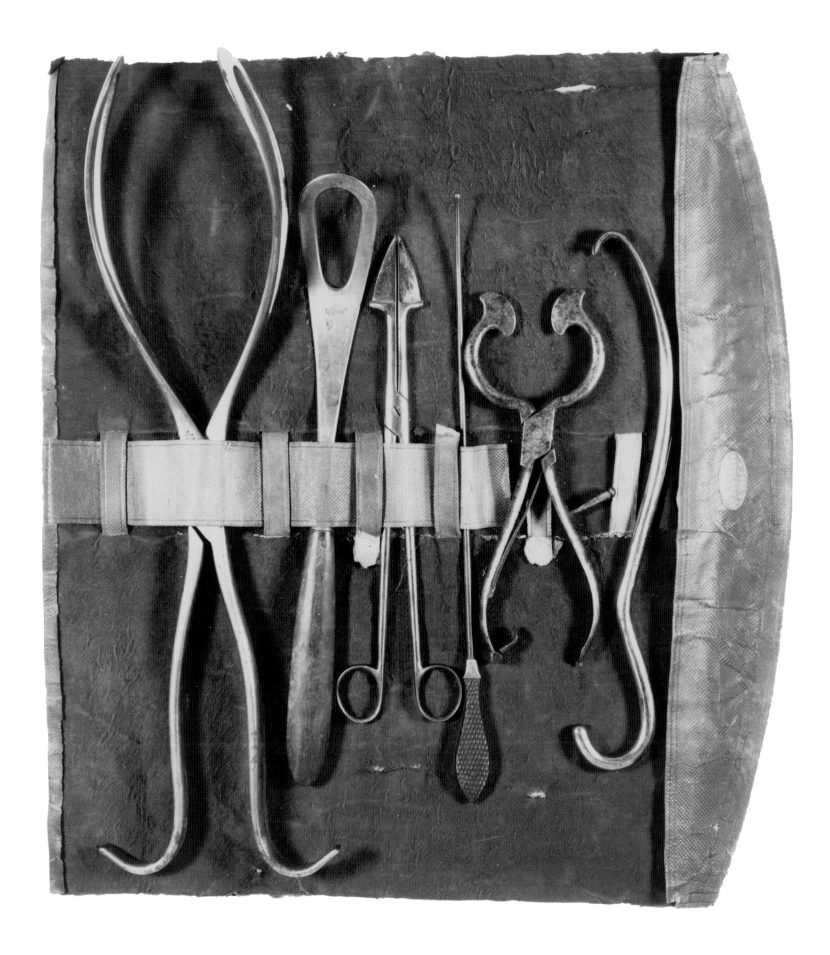

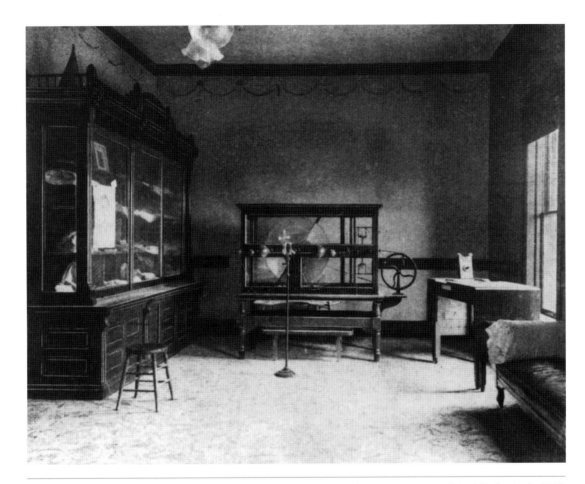

Left: Ohio physician John Richmond performed the first recorded cesarean section west of the Alleghenies in 1827 with "no recourse to cordials,...few medicines,...[and] only a case of common pocket instruments." His patient resumed work 24 days later. This later obstetrical kit offered its owner, Dr. Lewis Wolfley, a better selection of instruments with which to work.

Above: The discovery of x-rays by Wilhelm Roentgen in 1895 was one of the great medical breakthroughs of the century. Within a year, devices were in use in many countries. In 1899, an x-ray machine was installed at the A.T. Still Infirmary in Kirksville, Missouri, only the second such machine west of the Mississippi River.

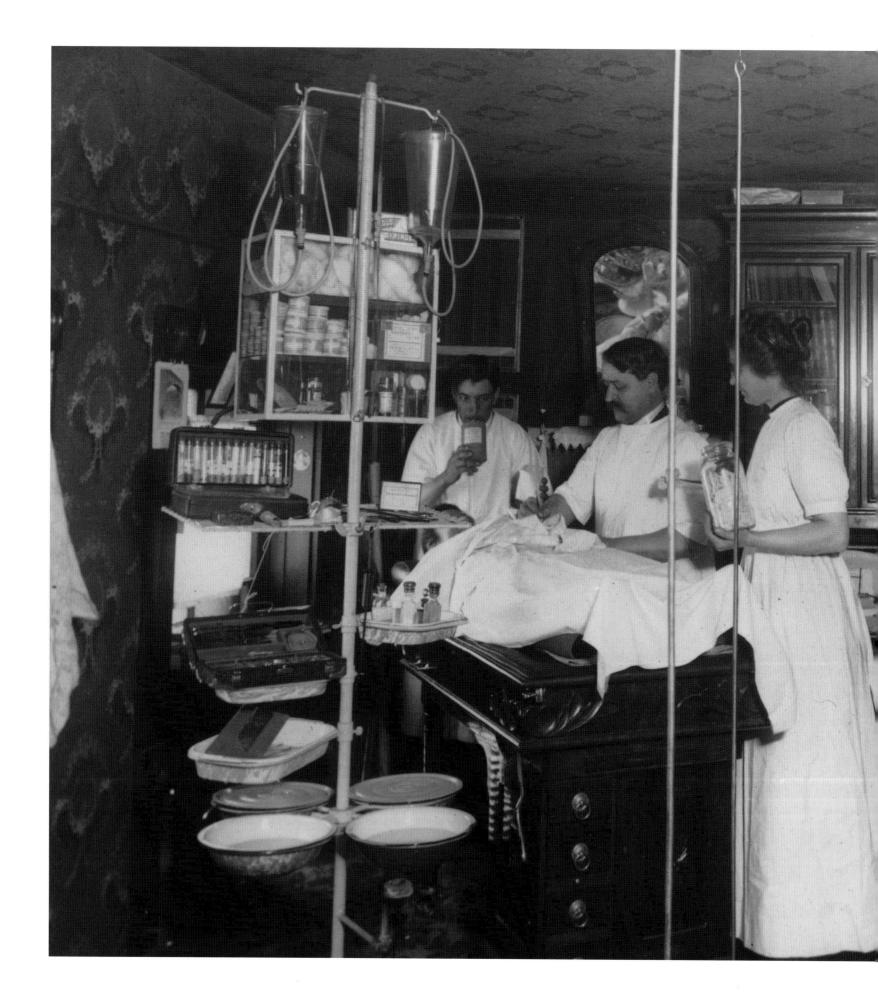

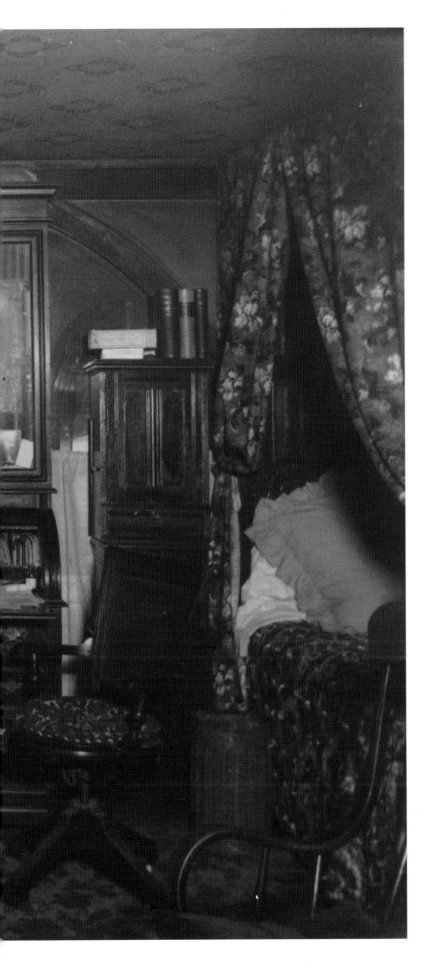

This carpeted and well-equipped office-surgery was atypical of the country practitioner. This unknown physician in Garden City, Kansas, was also especially fortunate to have a surgical assistant and nurse.

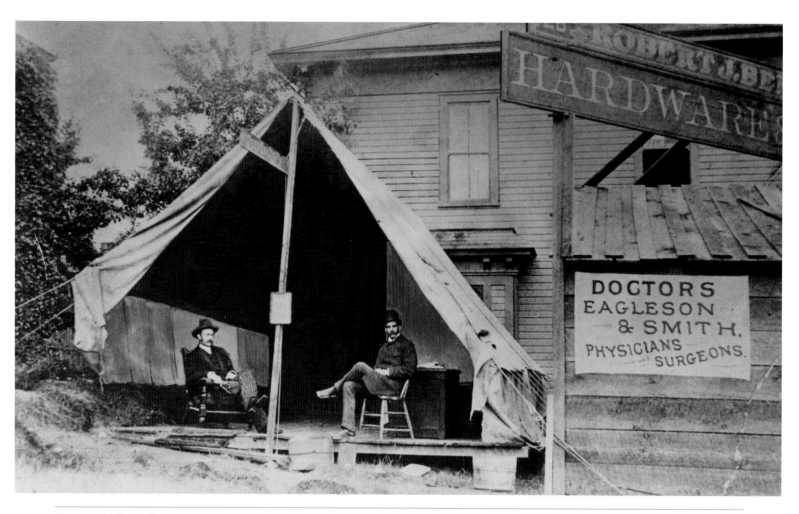

When an 1889 fire destroyed much of Seattle, Washington, Drs. Eagleson and Smith quickly reestablished their practice in improvised quarters.

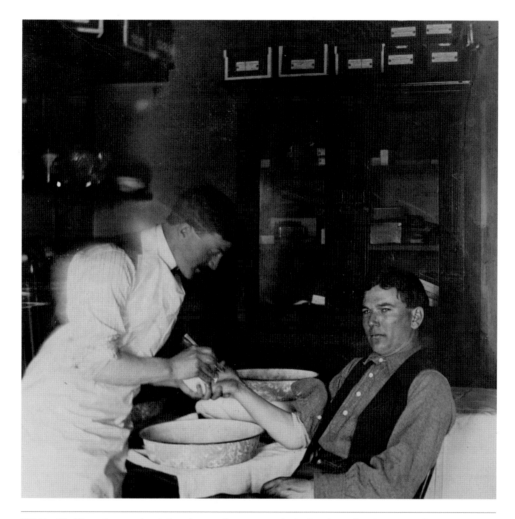

While this Wyoming cowboy's hand wound appears relatively minor, frontier town physicians were often called on to set broken bones from falls from horses, knife wounds, gunshot wounds, and cuts and abrasions from fights.

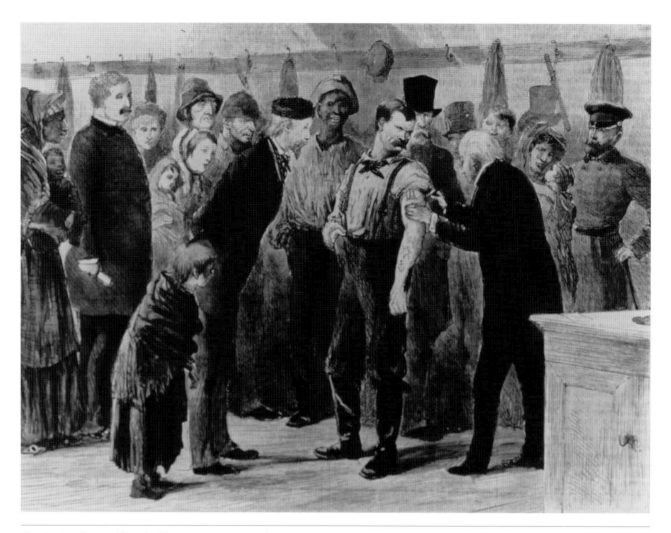

Vaccination for smallpox had been put into general use in 1800, but throughout the 19th century fear, apathy, and limited access to health care prevented its universal application. In the 1890s, some cities experienced violent protests as health officials attempted mass inoculation of immigrants.

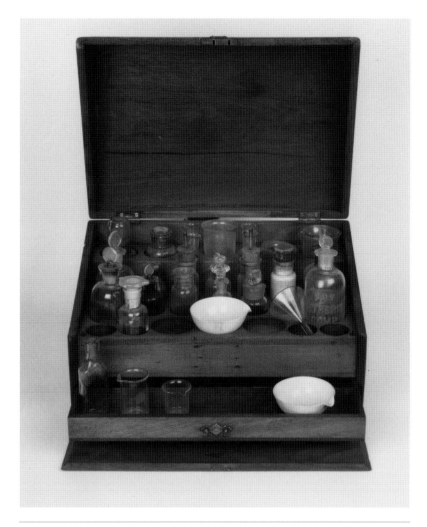

This portable office laboratory allowed physicians to carry out various diagnostic tests in their offices or the patients' homes.

STETHOSCOPES.

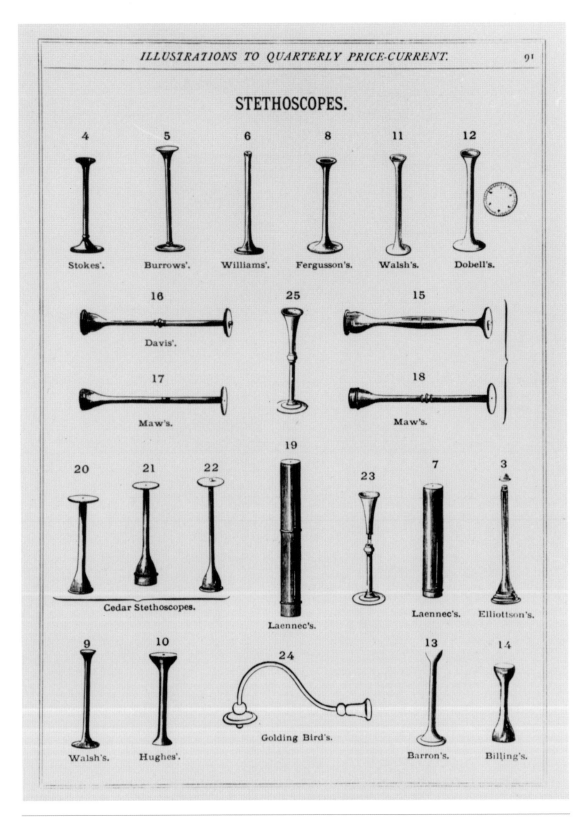

When Laennec introduced the stethoscope in 1819, he also provided a new terminology related to internal sounds and their relationship to disease. Practitioners either eagerly adopted this new diagnostic tool or warned of its dangers. Nevertheless, by the time this 1869 catalogue page appeared, monaural stethoscopes of various designs were widely in use.

CLINICAL THERMOMETERS.

Please Read and Carefully Observe these Directions.

Thermometers are in working order, and always ready for application when the top part of the small bit of mercury that forms the Index is below the arrow point. After using it, and in order to bring the Index again below the arrow point and ready for use, take the top part of the stem of the Thermometer (near the 105) between the thumb and first finger, with the bulb turned downward, or inclined toward the floor. In this position quietly swing from you (like a pendulum) from the elbow down, leave wrist hang as loose as possible. Always look at the position of your Index after each swing, until you again see the top part of it below the arrow point, and it is again ready for application. If it be found that one or two quiet swings is not sufficient to bring the top part of the Index below the arrow point let your swing be somewhat forcible. Don't shake the Index lower than is necessary.

One or more separations of the column does not put the instrument out of order. Always take the top part of the top separation for a reading, and so long as any separation remains the instrument is good for years.

By observing these directions you will have no trouble with your Thermometer.

FIG.		
*2892	Sharp & Smith's Self-Registering Indestructible Index Thermometer........................	$1 25
2893	Sharp & Smith's Self-Registering Indestructible Index Thermometer, black........................	1 50
*2894	Sharp & Smith's (Gilt Case and Chain) Self-Registering Indestructible Index Thermometer........................	1 75
*2895	Sharp & Smith's (one minute) Self-Registering Indestructible Index Thermometer........................	1 50
*2896	Hicks' Self-Registering Indestructible Index Thermometer.	1 50
2897	" Lens front " " " "	2 75
*2898	Spiral " " " "	1 25
*2899	T. & Co.'s Syphon " " " "	2 50
*2900	Spiral Surface Self-Registering Thermometer ....$6 00 to	7 50
2900A	Surface " " .... 2 50 to	7 50
*2901	Seguin's Surface " "	2 00

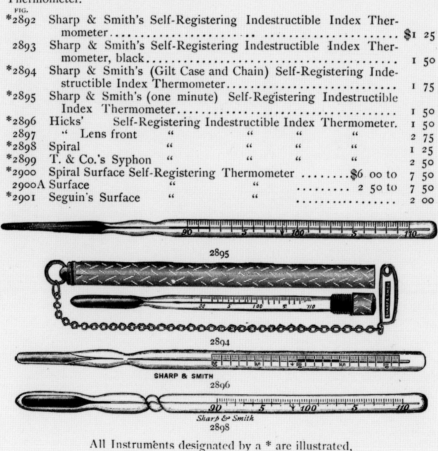

2895

2894

SHARP & SMITH
2896

Sharp & Smith
2898

All Instruments designated by a * are illustrated.

First developed in the 17th century, thermometers were slow to be accepted. For example, in 1867, American physicians imported fewer than 50 thermometers from England, but by 1876, more than 3000 had been purchased. The instrument's fragility, difficulties with calibration, the need for training in its use, and its lack of relationship to the prevailing local concept of disease contributed to physician resistance. By 1889, however, medical catalogues such as this one from Sharp and Smith offered various models and price ranges.

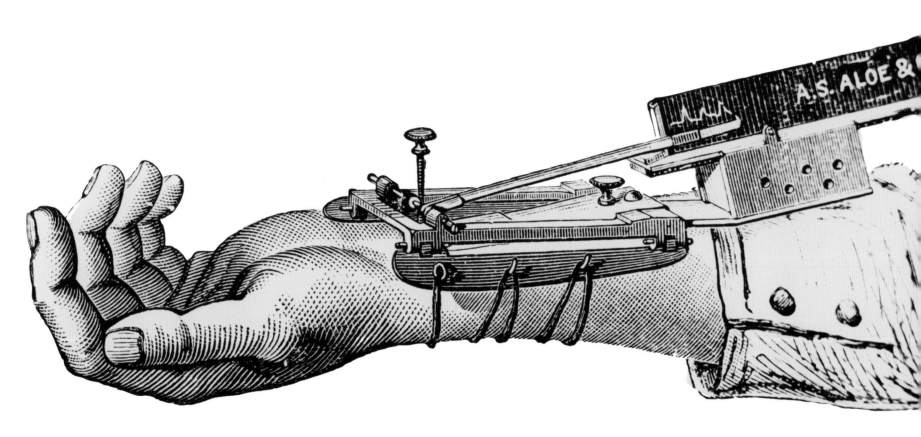

For over 2000 years the pulse had been seen as a basic sign of life and disease indicator. Not surprisingly, various attempts were made to quantify it. The first clinically useful sphygmograph was designed by Étienne Marey in 1860. As shown in this circa 1893 A.S. Aloe catalogue, it lay longitudinally on the forearm and provided a written record of arterial movement.

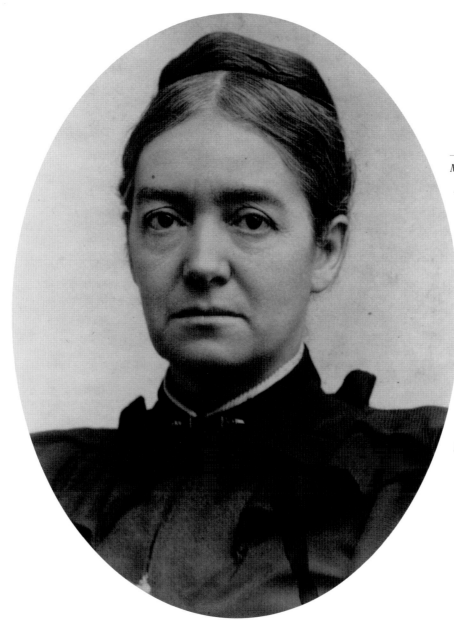

Mary Putnam Jacobi earned degrees from the New York College of Pharmacy, The Female Medical College of Pennsylvania, and the University of Paris. Submitting a paper anonymously, she won the highly competitive Boylston Medical Prize from Harvard. Teaching in two schools and writing, she also maintained an active private practice and, late in the 19th century, established a pioneering pediatric clinic at The Mount Sinai Hospital, New York, with her husband, Dr. Abraham Jacobi.

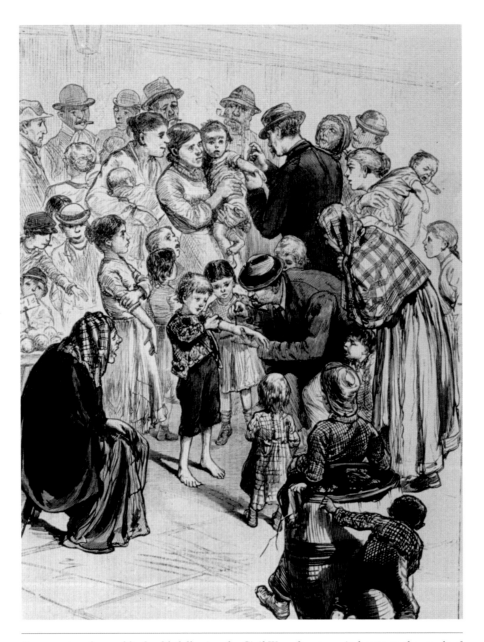

Progress in urban public health following the Civil War often came in bursts as the result of epidemics or other health scares. For example, in Jersey City, New Jersey, a smallpox scare brought about compulsory inoculation of all citizens, including the poorest slum dwellers.

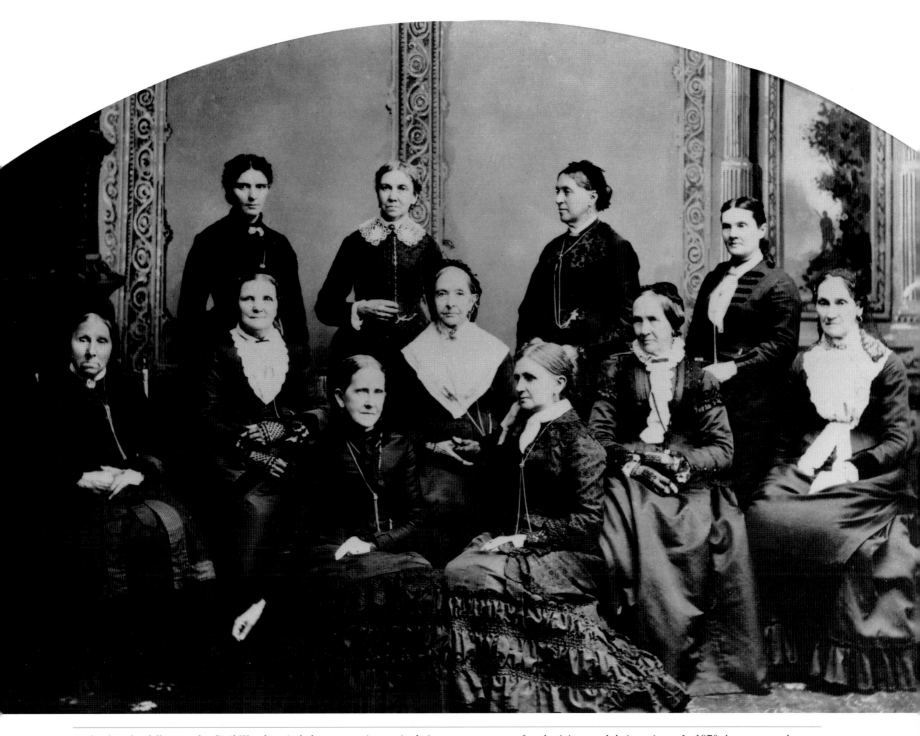

In the decades following the Civil War, hospitals became an increasingly important resource for physicians and their patients. In 1870 there were only about 100 hospitals nationwide, but within the next 50 years, nearly 6000 would be built. In 1882 the women of the Mormon Relief Society founded Deseret Hospital. Among them were Dr. Ellis Reynolds Shipp, standing left, and Dr. Romania Pratt Penrose, standing right, the first female physician in Utah.

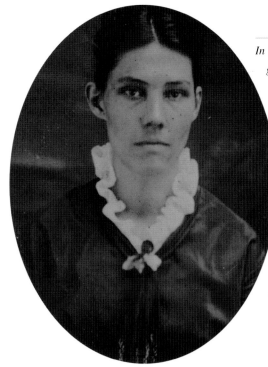

In 1849 the first medical degree was granted to a woman, Elizabeth Blackwell, by the Geneva (New York) Medical College. By 1870 about 600 women were practicing medicine, although many had gotten their education at homeo- pathic, eclectic, and other "irregular" medical schools. Dr. Georgia Arbuckle Fix established an active practice in Nebraska in the fourth quarter of the 19th century.

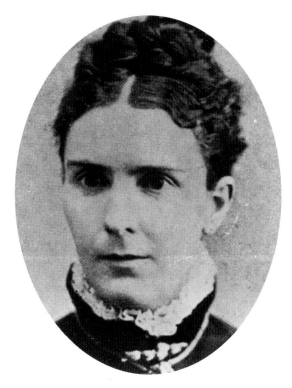

Dr. Ellis Reynolds Shipp maintained a practice, served on the Deseret (Utah) Hospital board, and headed a nurses home that graduated 500 women.

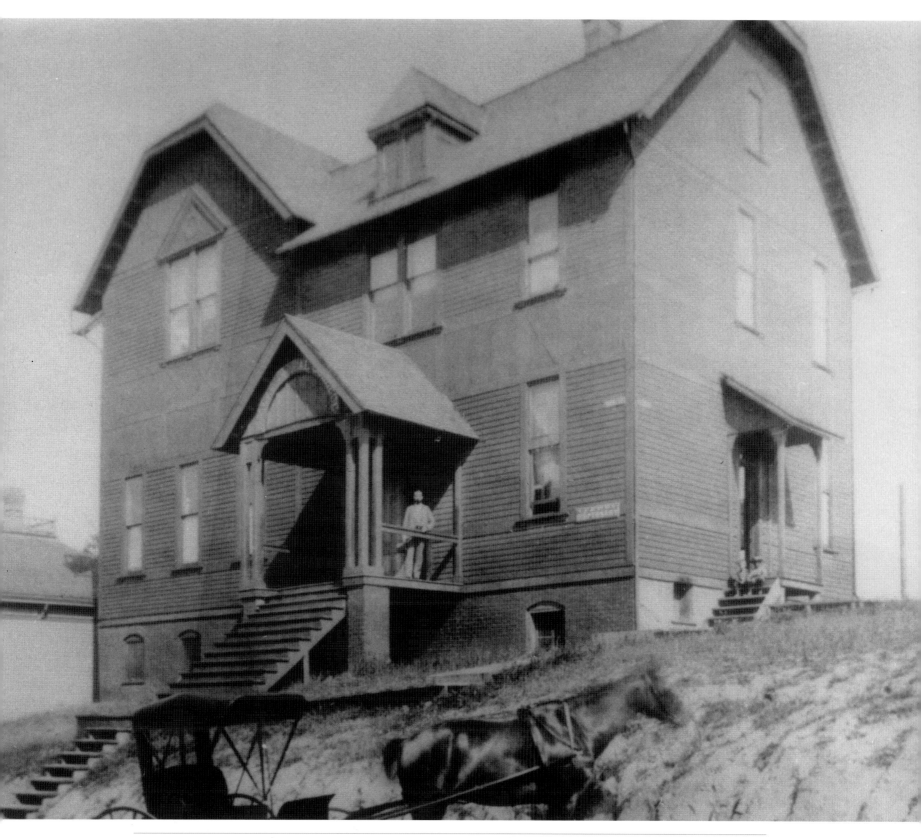

The Omaha Medical College as it appeared in 1887. During the period between 1875 and 1890, nearly 100 medical schools would be opened, many to meet the demands for frontier physicians. The program largely consisted of four-month terms, with exactly the same classes taken two consecutive years. It wasn't until the end of the century that major changes were widely instituted, requiring an entrance examination, a six- to nine-month school year, a three-year program, and written and oral course examinations.

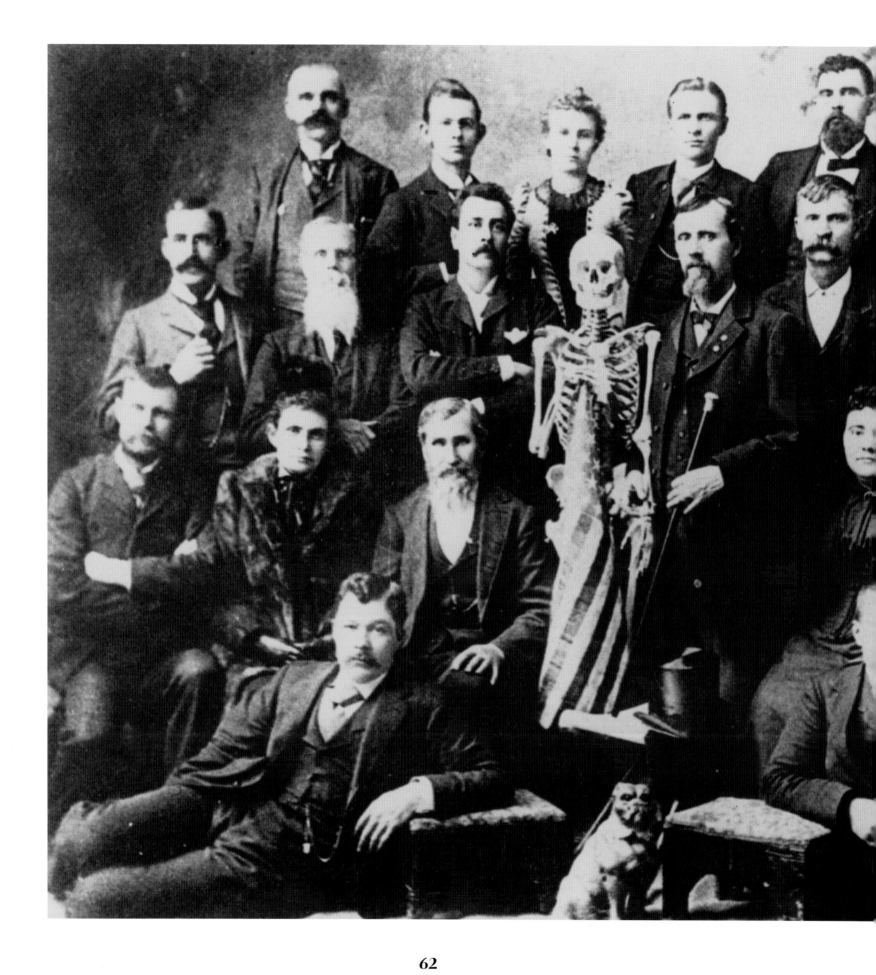

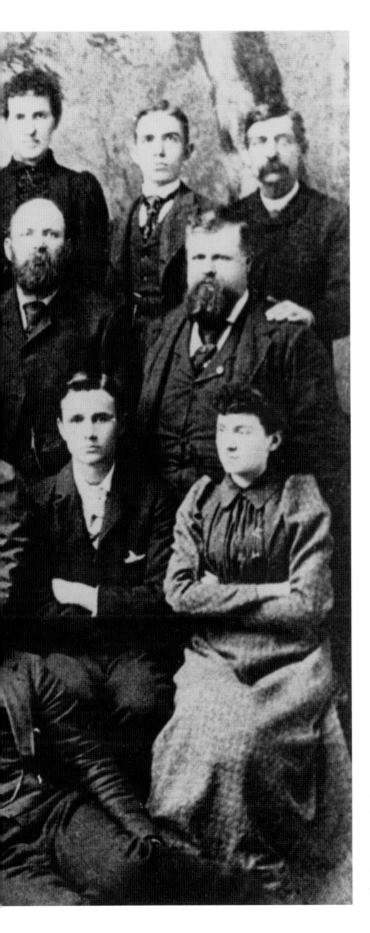

In 1892 Dr. Andrew Taylor Still (center with stick) founded the American School of Osteopathy in Kirksville, Missouri, to teach the alternative form of medicine he had formulated just three years before. The men and women in this first graduating class would join homeopaths, hydrotherapists, eclectics, Mesmerists, and practitioners of a dozen other "irregular" philosophies that flourished in the largely unregulated Western frontier. Unlike most of these alternatives, however, osteopathy continues today alongside allopathic medicine.

Chapter 4

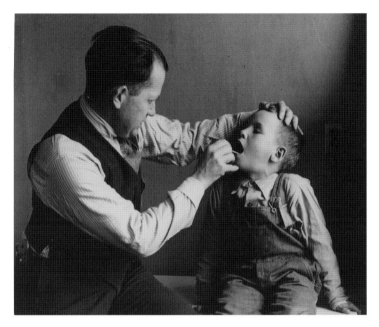

ONE AMONG MANY
1901–1945

The 20th century would see medicine move its focus away from the solo practitioner and his or her black bag. The family physician was becoming part of a system.

One element of this system that would assume dominance, at least for a while, was the hospital. No longer akin to workhouses or simply a place where the poor went to die, hospitals prospered from the benefits of pain-free surgery; decreased infection rates; developments in laboratory analysis, x-ray and other technology; and improved nursing and management techniques. Both patients and physicians seemed eager to transfer the locus of care to these facilities.

In the hospital, patients received care from a growing variety of professionals. General physicians were joined by trained nurses, laboratory technicians, surgeons, pathologists, x-ray technicians, and an increasing number of medical specialists. Medical education put interns and residents at the bedside. Elite hospitals even maintained research laboratories.

Government, too, would assume an ever-greater role in this medical system. In the cities east of the Mississippi, infrastructure building projects attempted to keep up with population growth. Improved sanitation, municipal health departments, and requirements for reporting contagious diseases helped to control epidemics and improve the general environment for city dwellers.

Improvements lagged behind in rural and western areas. Efforts at the federal level, first with expansion of the responsibilities of the Public Health Service and then with the creation of the Depression-era Farm Security Administration, would eventually bring developments in sanitation and health care services to these underserved areas. Additional federal activities that established the Veterans Administration and the National Institutes of Health, among others, would ensure a role for the federal government in both medical care and research for the foreseeable future.

Right: As the 20th century began, American physicians remained primarily general practitioners in solo practice. They cared for their patients in an office or at the bedside, but only the poorest patients went to hospitals. This posed photograph, probably staged by photographer W.H. Willard Jones in Chicago around the turn of the century, is an idealized version of the solo practitioner.

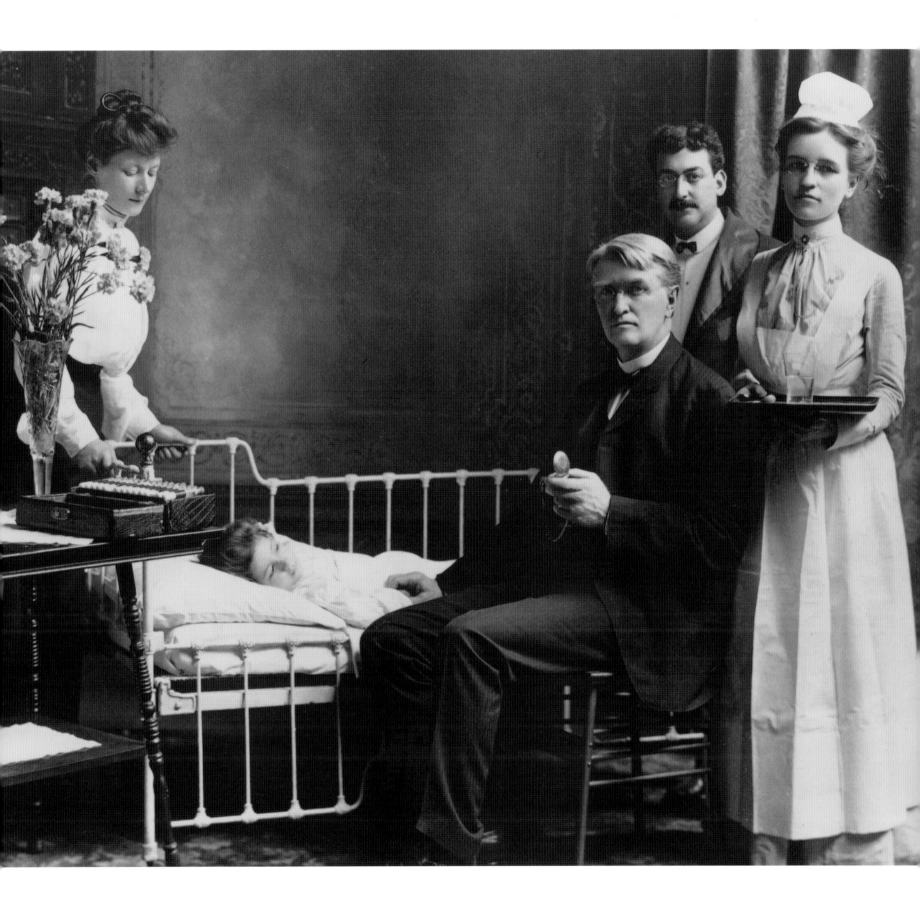

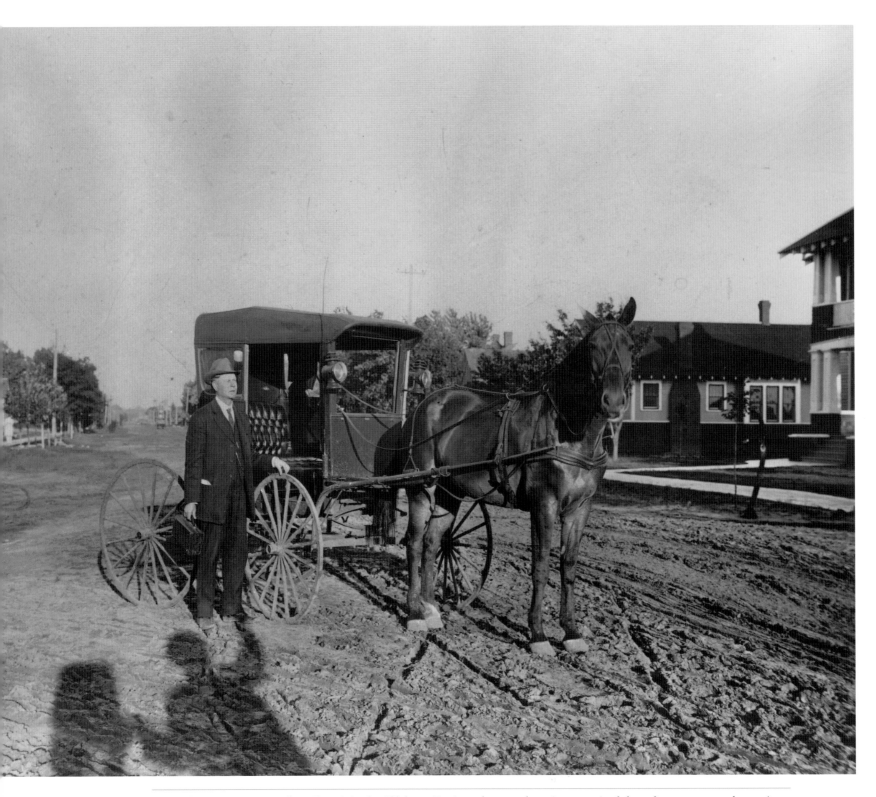

On the frontier, in towns such as Francis in the Oklahoma Territory, horse and carriage remained the safest way to travel to patients. Paved roads were nonexistent, and distances between homes meant long hikes for frequently stranded travellers.

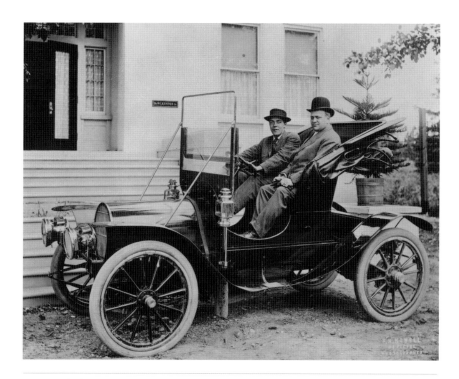

Despite the hazards dirt roads posed, many physicians were among the first in their communities to purchase automobiles. In Seattle, Washington, for example, Dr. Rininger (derby hat) owned the third automobile in the city. In some cases, doctors retained their horse and carriage for country or night calls and used their automobile for town travel.

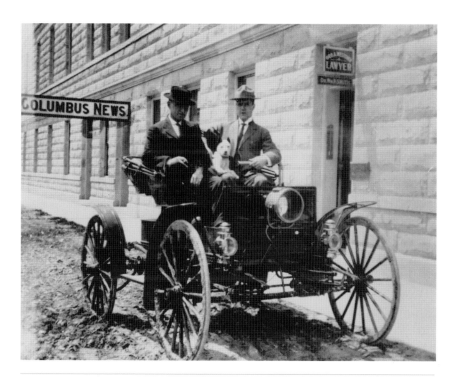

Dr. William Smith braved the dirt roads of Columbus, Montana, in a tiller-steered high wheeler. Not surprisingly, many physicians were vocal advocates for paved roads. Dr. William Higgins, for example, was elected in the 1930s to his state senate with the motto "Get Connecticut Out of the Mud."

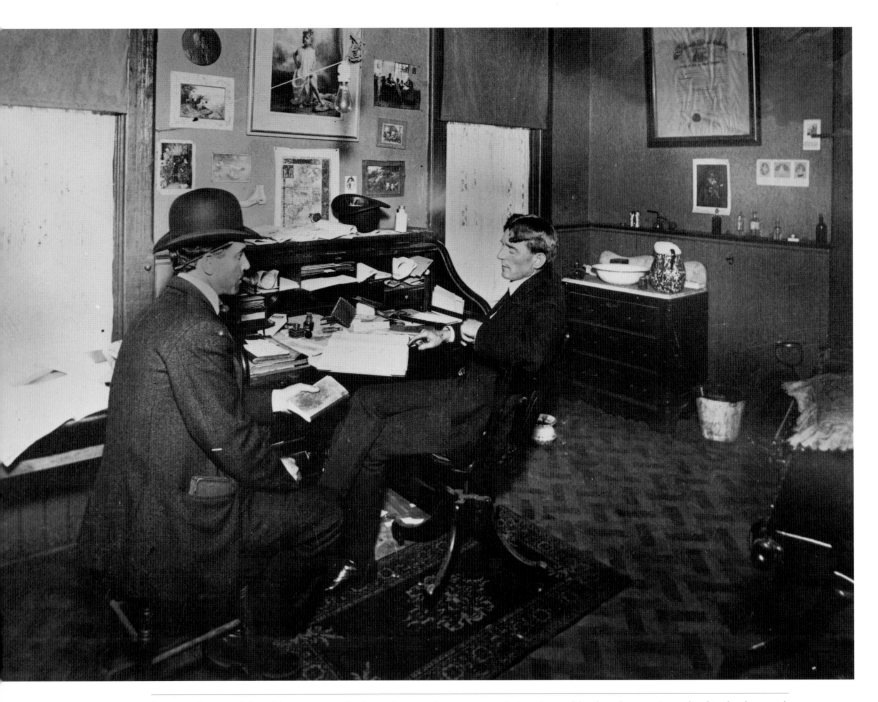

In the early part of the 20th century, medical practice in urban areas was being changed by the advances in medical technology and science. However, in rural and frontier America, physicians could seldom turn to x-ray machines or laboratories. Dr. T.S. Chapman's office in McAlester, Oklahoma, could boast of electricity but no running water.

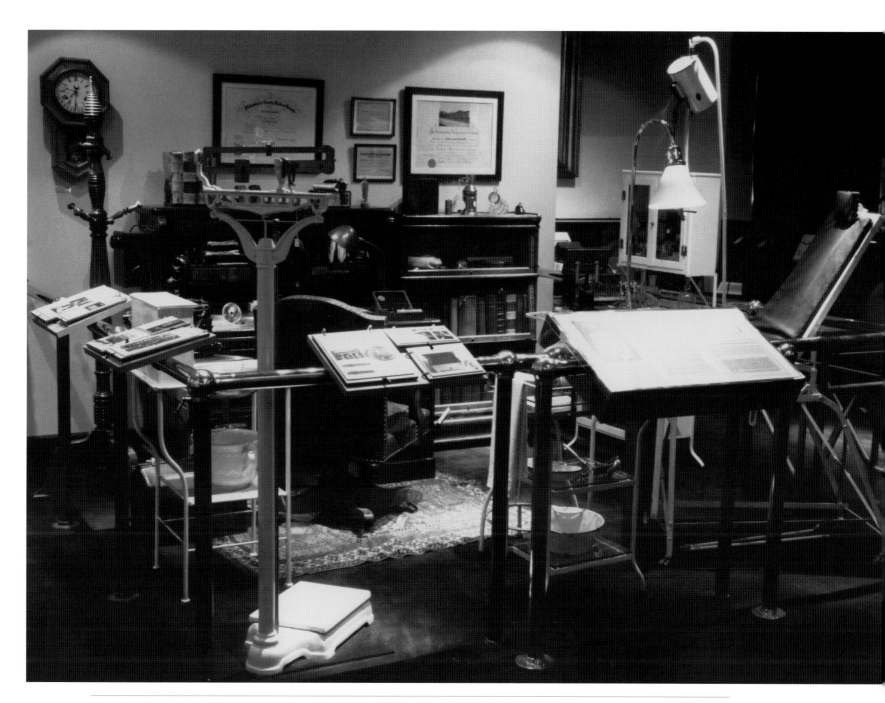

When Dr. Philip Gordon Kitchen set up his suburban Philadelphia office in 1911 (re-created here), he could install many of the latest devices, including a flexible examining table, telephone, sphygmomanometer, and electricity. Yet, like the Oklahoma physician in the previous photograph, Dr. Kitchen also did not have running water for his use.

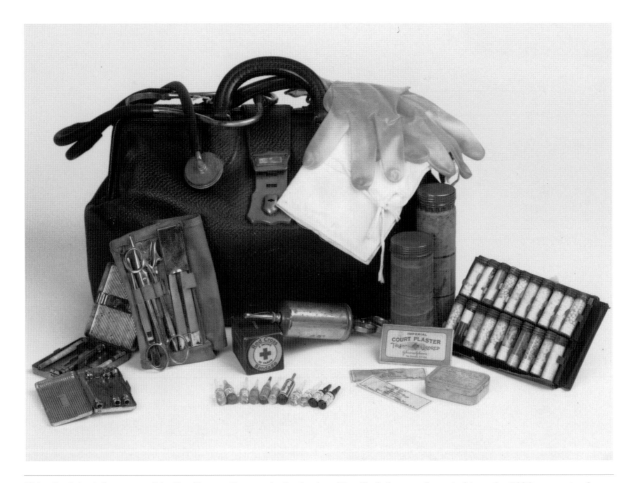

This physician's bag, owned by Dr. George Comstock of suburban New York State and carried into the 1920s, contained everything needed to deal with most common illnesses and minor injuries: syringe case, surgical kit, ampules of medications, and a tablet case of commonly prescribed pills.

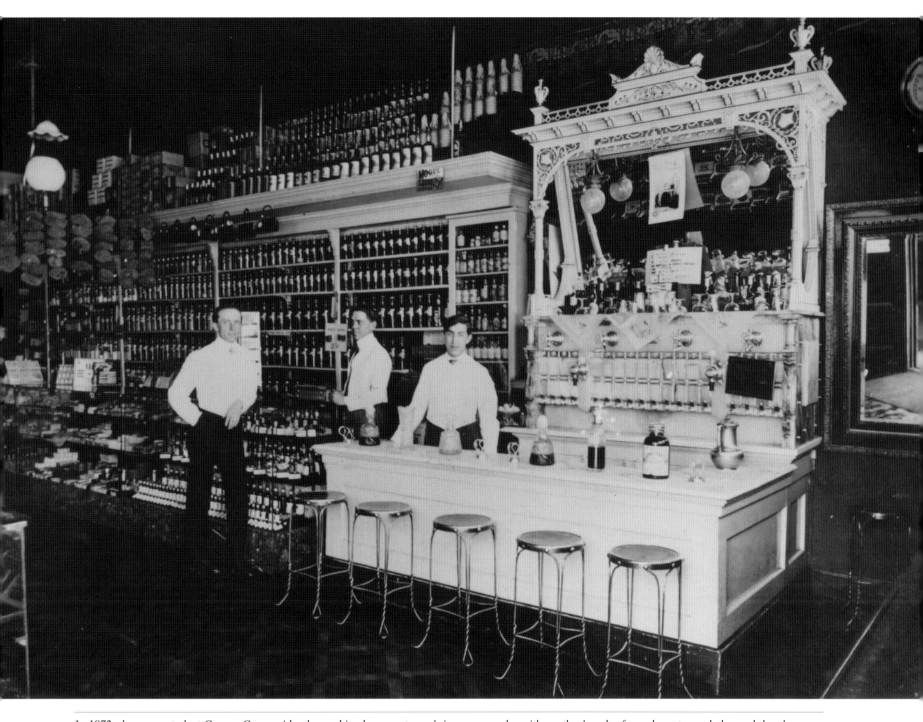

In 1872 pharmacy student George Guy accidently combined one customer's ice cream order with another's order for soda water and changed the pharmacy forever. The soda fountain, such as this ornate one in Moritz Drugstore, Denver, Colorado, in 1906, quickly replaced a chair next to the potbellied stove as the place for locals to gather and chat.

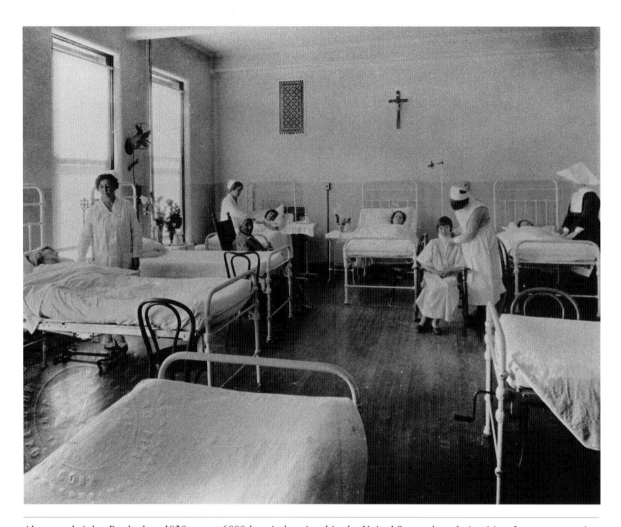

Above and right: By the late 1920s, over 6000 hospitals existed in the United States, largely in cities. Improvements in cleanliness, professionalism of nurses, and developments such as anesthesia and antisepsis all contributed to improving the image of hospitals, especially among the upper and middle classes. Note that while the sexes were segregated in women's and men's wards, children and adults were not.

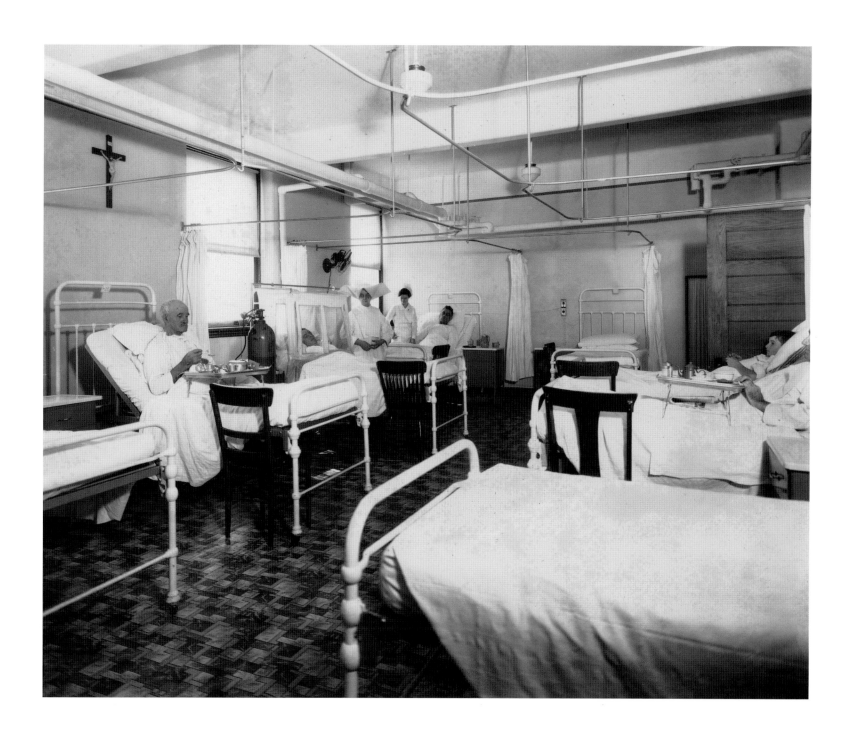

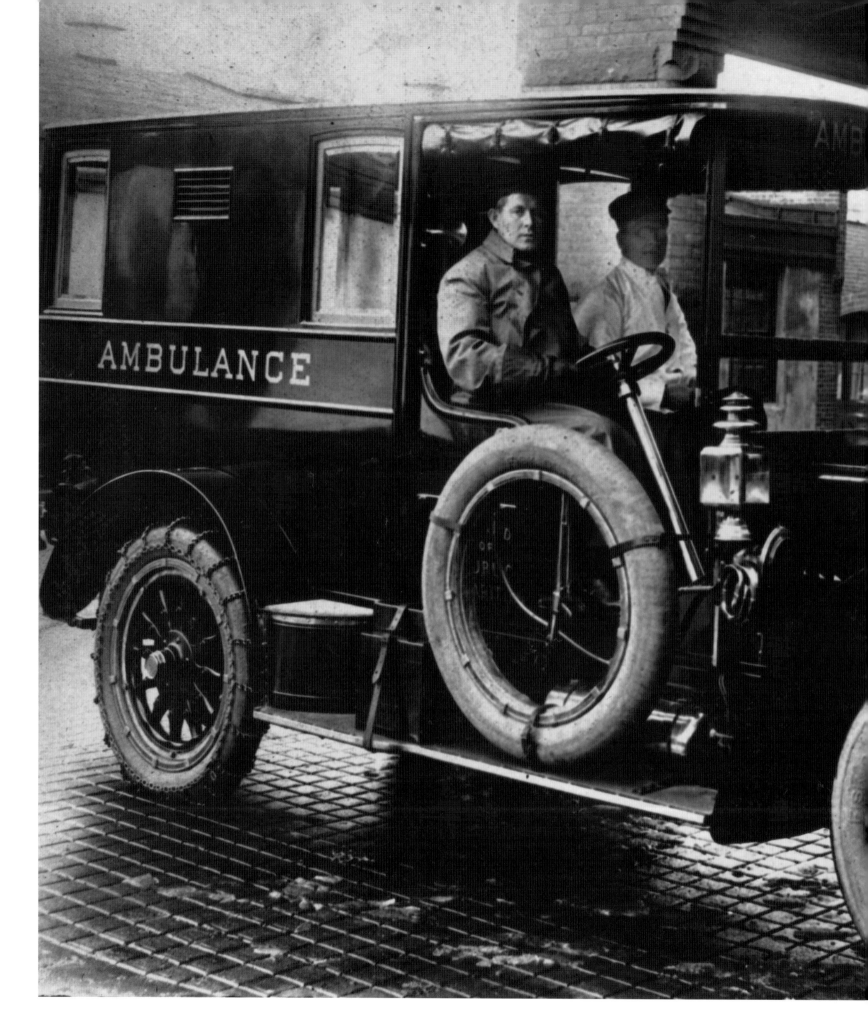

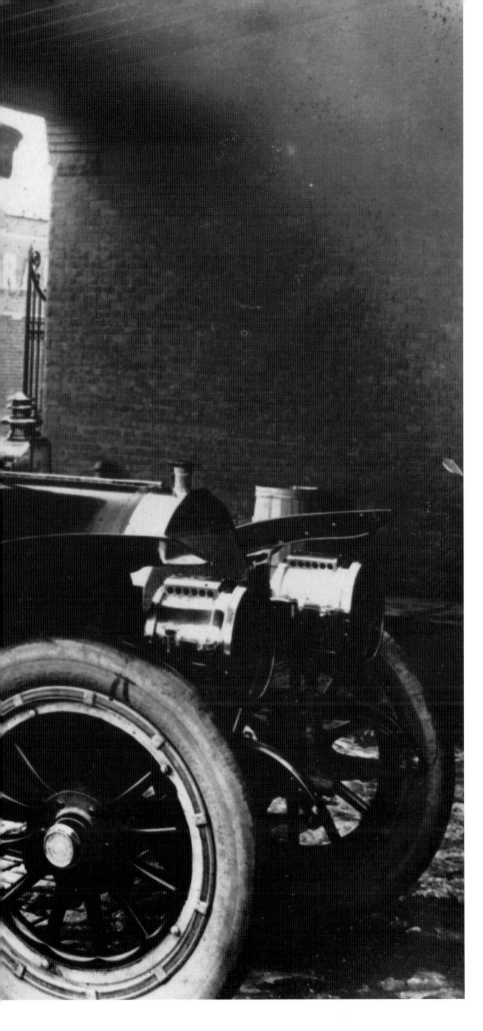

As the number of people treated in hospitals rose, so did the need for fast transportation to carry the most seriously ill patients to these institutions. This 1909 Locomobile ambulance was the first motor-driven ambulance in Bridgeport, Connecticut.

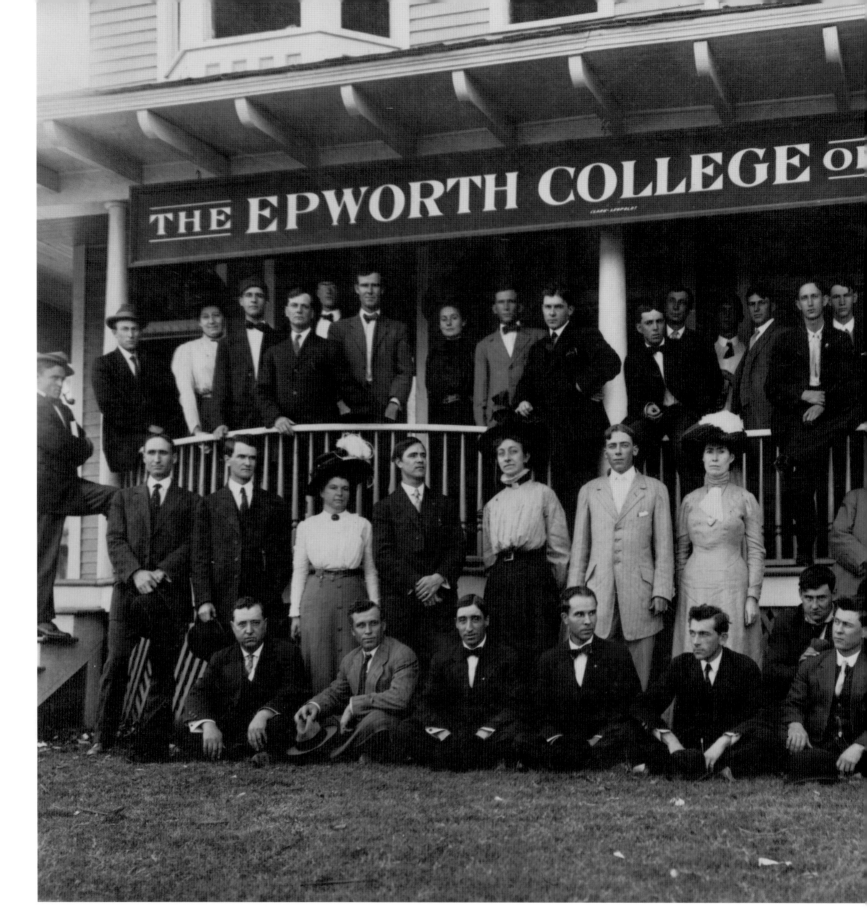

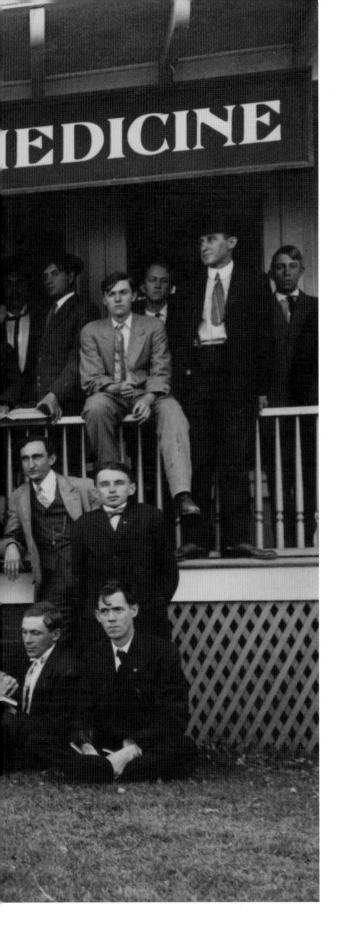

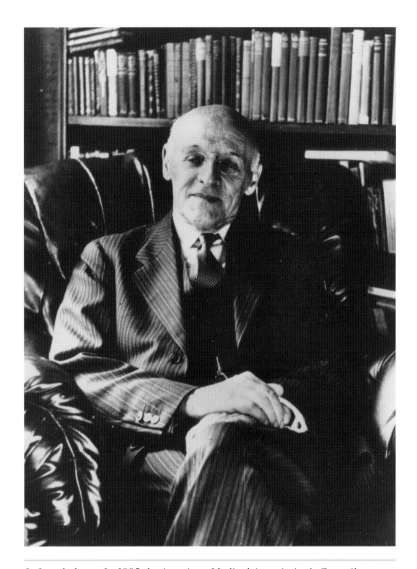

Left and above: In 1905 the American Medical Association's Council on Medical Education recommended as an "ideal standard" for medical education that students have a high-school education followed by four years of medical school and one year of internship. However, it wasn't until Abraham Flexner's report on medical education in the United States and Canada five years later that significant reform began.

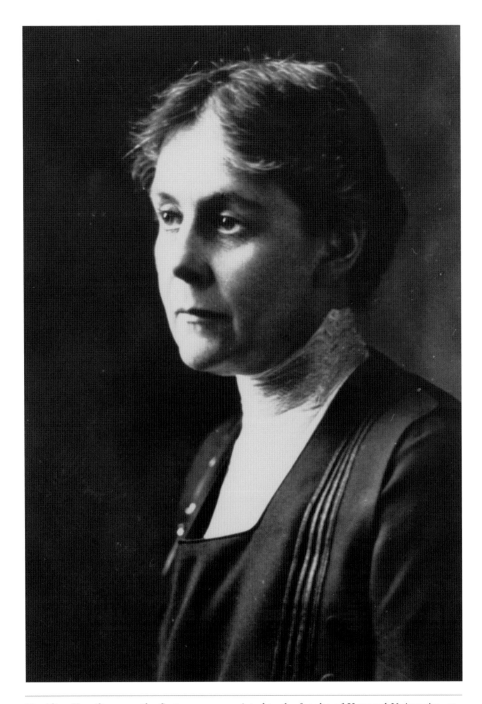

Dr. Alice Hamilton was the first woman appointed to the faculty of Harvard University, at a time when women were still not admitted to the medical school. Although her interest in occupational medicine would eventually take her away from direct patient care, she spent her early career at Hull House, the well-known Chicago settlement house where she set up the first well-baby clinic in the United States and saw first-hand the immense health toll modern industry was taking on its workers. As the result of her efforts, Illinois passed the first Workmen's Compensation Act that included both industrial illness and injury.

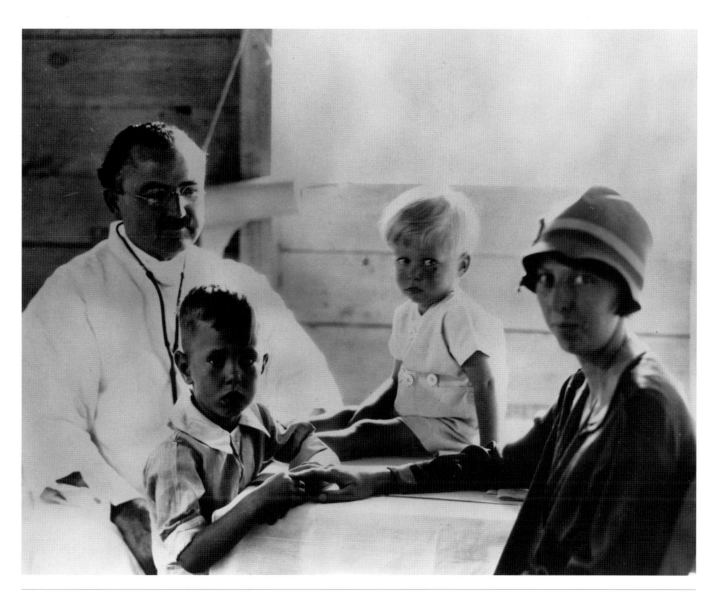

In the early 1930s only one half of the U.S. population visited a physician within a given year, with the number of visits averaging 2.6 per person annually. Fifty years later, the number of visits would increase by over 40% and four of five Americans would visit a doctor each year.

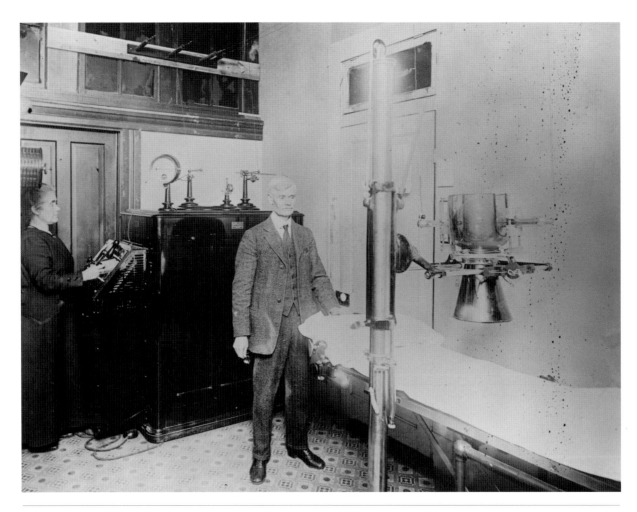

X-ray technology was quickly accepted by the medical profession, and fast-paced developments in x-ray diagnosis only served to increase enthusiasm. In 1916 Dr. Alexander Barkley set up what was probably the first x-ray machine in Oklahoma in his Harbart office. The discovery at the turn of the century of radiopaque suspensions to increase gastrointestinal tract visibility plus refinements in the x-ray equipment itself meant tumors could be identified at early stages, tuberculosis could be diagnosed early, and a patient's inner processes could be examined without risky surgery.

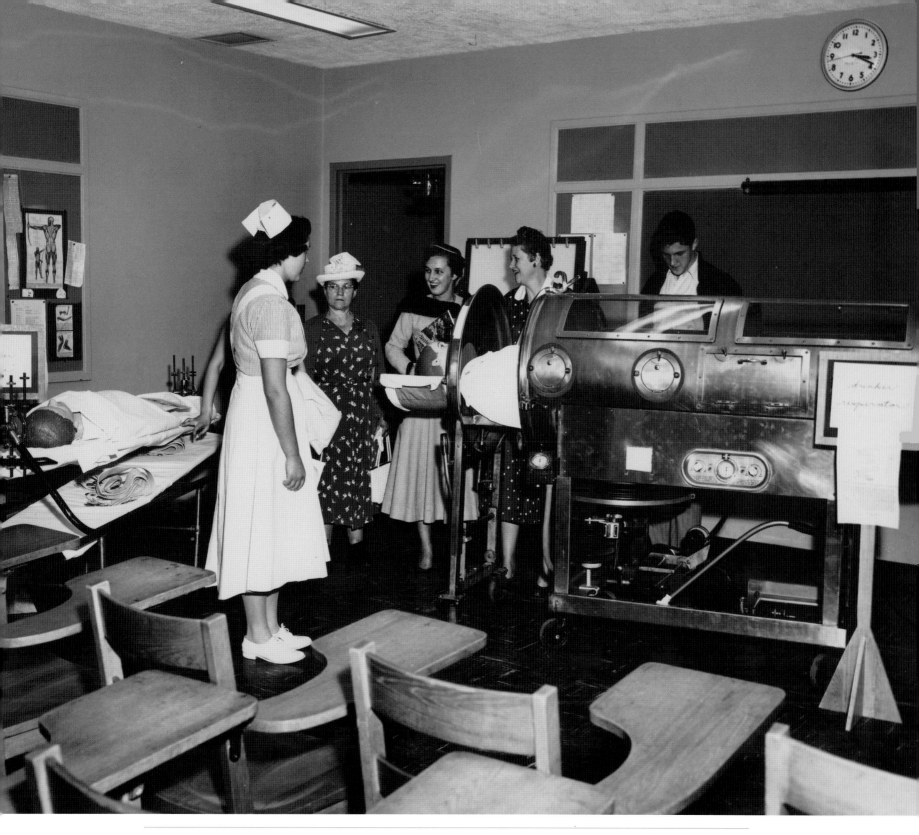

Diseases that struck children in large numbers were particularly devastating to parents and physicians alike. By World War II, diphtheria, whooping cough, and scarlet fever were or soon would be under control. Poliomyelitis, on the other hand, seemed able to attack at will without any medical recourse. In 1928 the iron lung was invented to ease breathing in polio victims.

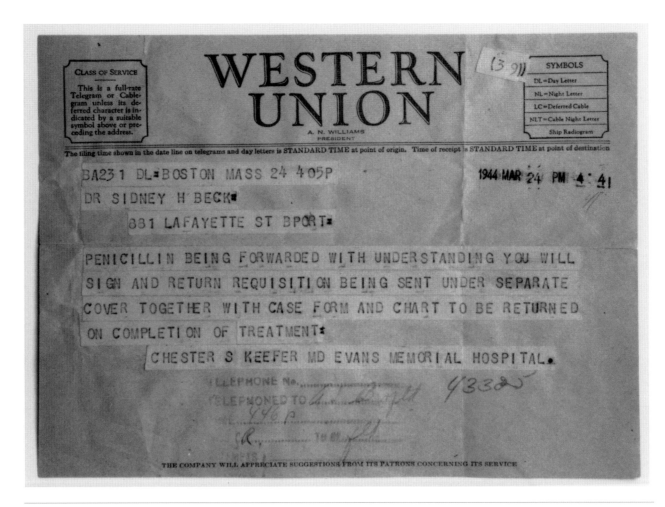

Above: In 1941 British researchers Howard Florey and Ernst Chain identified the therapeutic value of penicillin as an antibacterial agent. Yet as World War II reached its peak, production of penicillin lagged behind demand. As a result, civilian use was rigidly controlled. This 1944 telegram authorized what was probably the drug's first use in Bridgeport, Connecticut, for a 22-year-old man who was seriously ill with gonorrhea.

Right: During the Depression the Farm Security Administration offered prepaid health care plans directed toward low-income farm families and migrant workers. Services were provided in doctors' offices, in patients' homes, and in clinics such as the one in Reedsville, West Virginia, where this photograph was taken. At their height, FSA plans had 600 000 enrollees, along with providing clinic care for 150 000 migratory workers and their families.

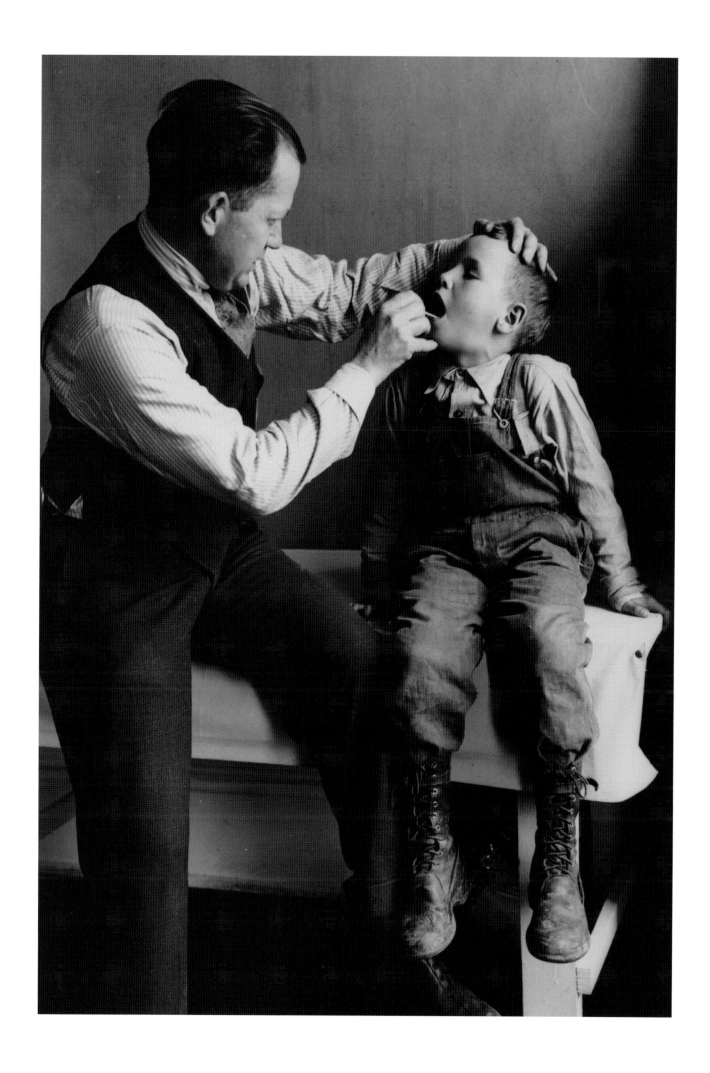

Chapter 5

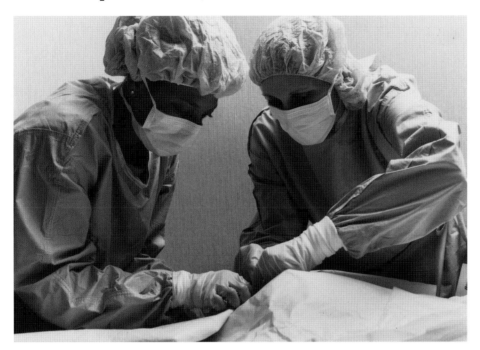

THE PHYSICIAN AS COORDINATOR 1946–PRESENT

By the second half of the 20th century, America's physicians were able to prevent or cure many of the contagious diseases that had once carried off younger patients—diphtheria, cholera, yellow fever, and smallpox, among them. While other diseases, such as AIDS and Legionnaires' disease, would take their place, nevertheless overall life expectancy rose significantly. The 1990 census recorded 248.7 million Americans, 12 percent of whom were over 65 years of age.

With increasing numbers of older patients, contemporary physicians face new epidemics of degenerative diseases—heart disease, cancer, stroke, kidney failure, and Alzheimer's disease. While billions of dollars are spent for research into cures and therapies, family physicians, in particular, find themselves drawn into renewed efforts at prevention and wellness.

Family physicians also find themselves at the heart of a managed care system that is significantly changing the way Americans receive care. An estimated 149 million Americans were enrolled in health maintenance organizations and preferred provider organizations in 1995. This system, with its reliance on family physicians and other primary care providers as care coordinators, has refocused attention on the value of family physicians as managers of health care. When family practice was established as a specialty in 1969, the "Essentials for Residency Training in Family Practice" included family medicine, internal medicine, pediatrics, psychiatry, obstetrics/gynecology, surgery, and community medicine. Such broad-based training enables family physicians to offer comprehensive, high-quality health care.

By the second half of this century, medical science seemed to have control over many communicable diseases. Polio was not one of them. In 1952 a polio epidemic affected 50 000 Americans—mostly children—and killed 3300 persons. Others were left with lungs so incapacitated by the virus that an iron lung was needed to help them breathe. Just three years later, the Salk vaccine was successfully tested, and polio vaccinations became standard procedure for family doctors and their patients. In 1960 Dr. Albert Sabin developed an oral liquid polio vaccine, and scenes such as this one at Los Angeles County Hospital became a part of history.

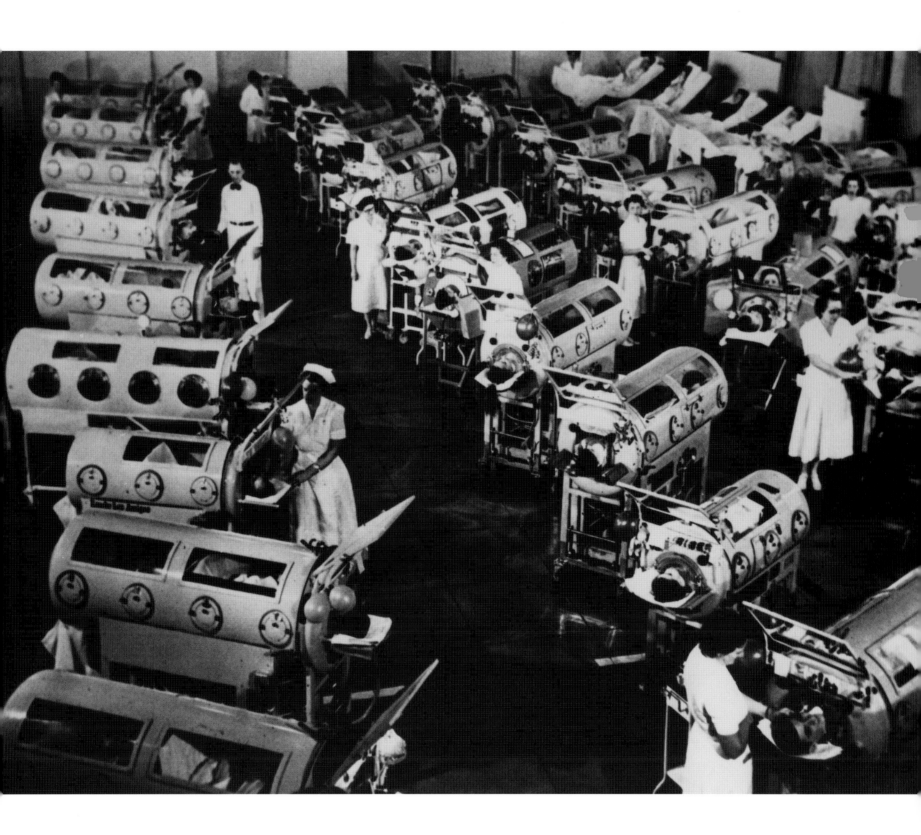

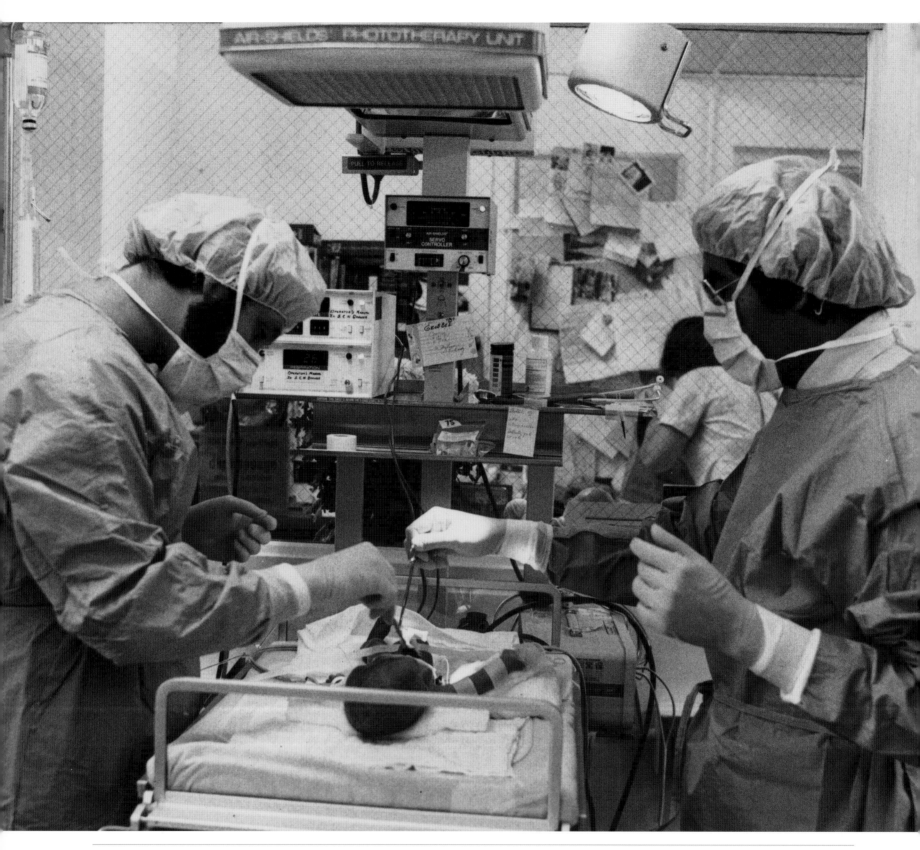

Neonatal mortality has dropped to one quarter the rate of the late 1940s for various reasons, not the least of which is the technologically advanced Neonatal Intensive Care Unit.

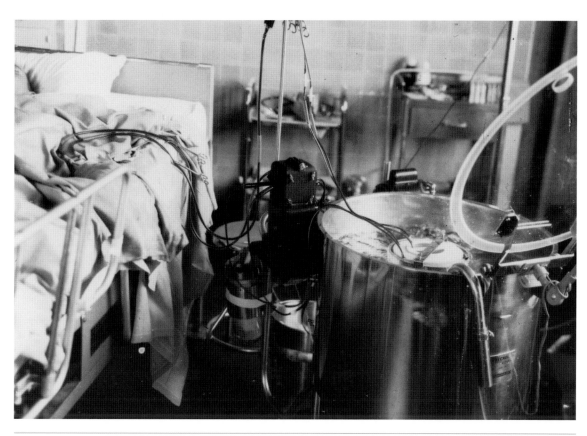

In 1945 the first kidney dialysis machine was available for use with patients. Various modifications aimed at simplifying the process and making the devices smaller were undertaken, and by the 1950s machines such as this one made their way into community hospitals. Today's devices enable patients to undergo dialysis at home, usually while awaiting a kidney transplant.

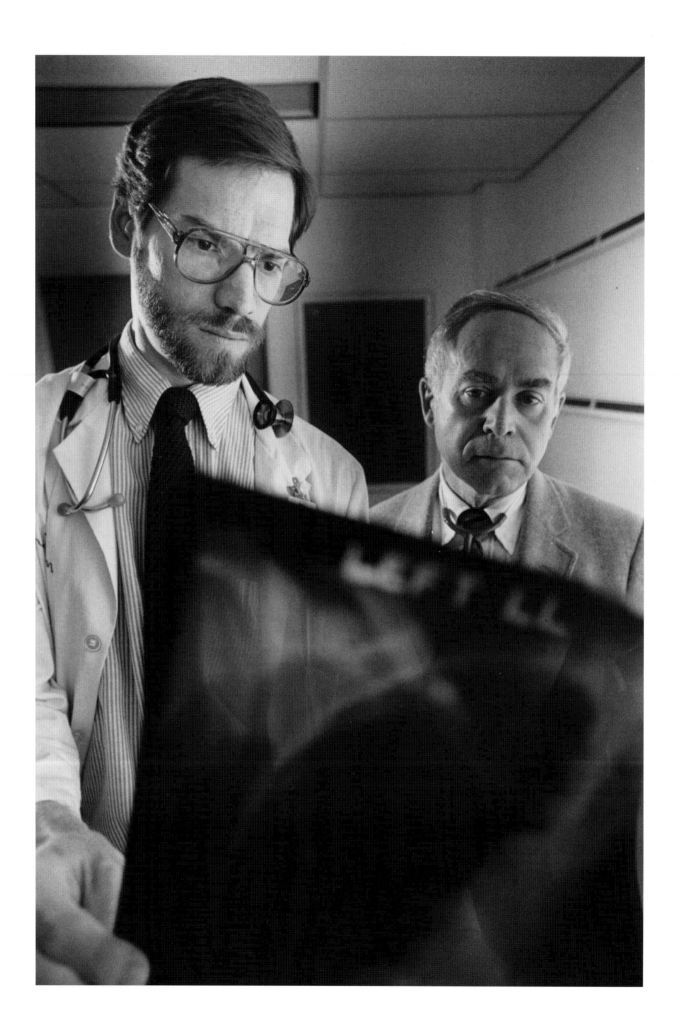

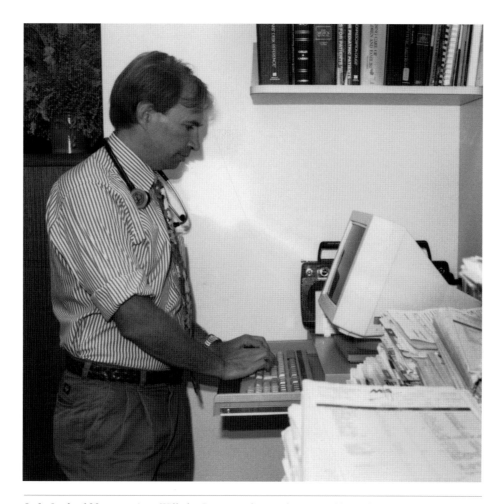

Left: In the 100 years since Wilhelm Roentgen first took x-rays of his wife's hand, developments in radiologic and other imaging techniques have advanced the physician's ability to diagnose disease. Nuclear scans, ultrasound, angiography, magnetic resonance imaging, and computerized tomography can show details of soft tissues, blood vessels, and cross sections of all parts of the body, respectively. This is far removed from the 17th-century diagnosis based on an "examination" of a fully clothed patient.

Above: The ubiquitous computer revolution of the final two decades of the 20th century has made itself felt in the physician's office as well. Electronic claims processing, computerized medical records, diagnostic scenario software, Internet access to medical databases throughout the world, and computerized literature searches are some of the more common ways in which computers are enhancing medical practice. In addition, especially in rural areas, computerized links to major medical centers provide access to specialists and specialty facilities for all patients.

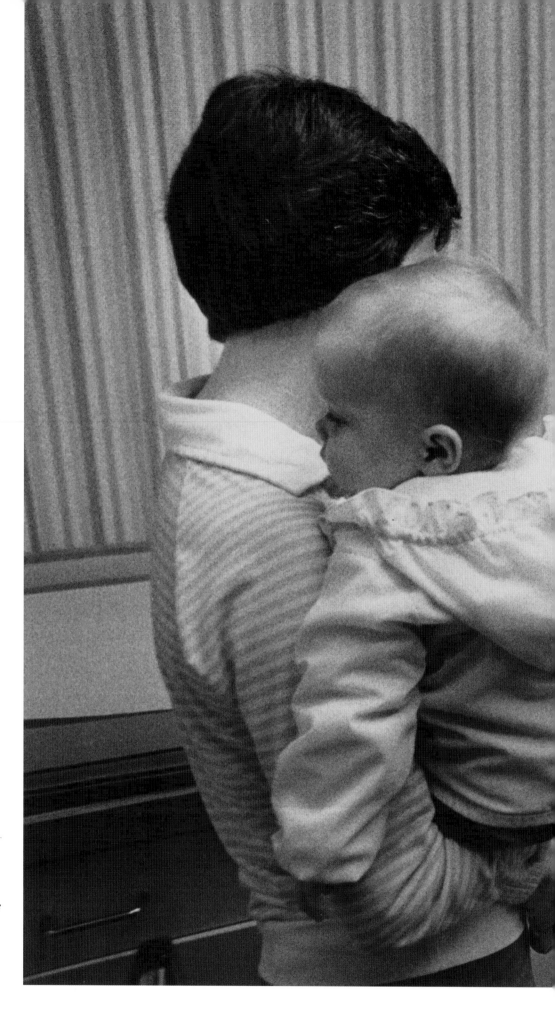

*In 1969 family practice was established as the 20th
certified specialty. From the beginning, the Family
Practice Unit/Center has been integral to residency
training programs. Residents are responsible for the care
of increasing numbers of patients over the three-year
training period. Unlike their 17th-century predecessors,
today's physicians will have seen and cared for many
patients of all ages before setting up practice.*

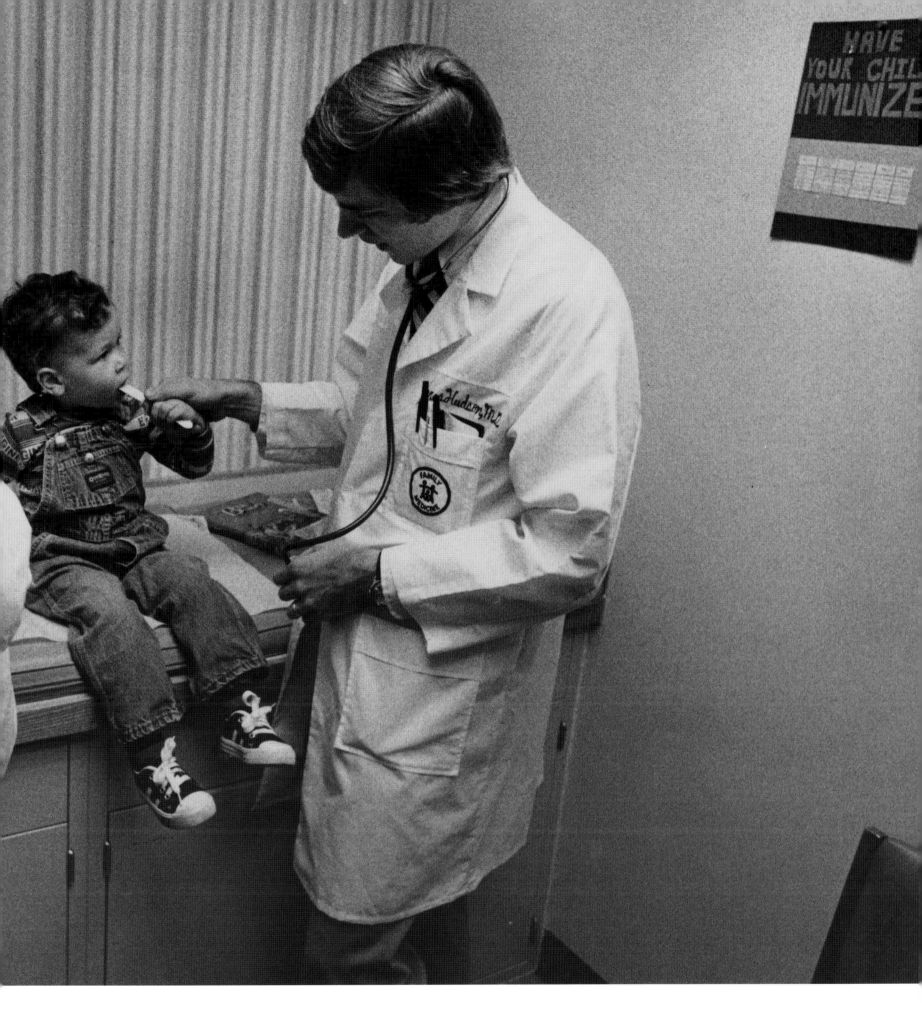

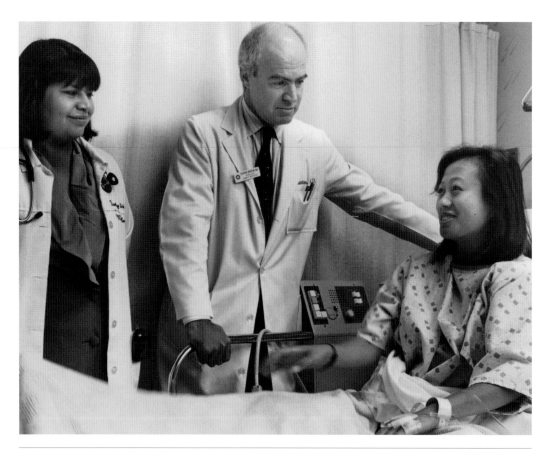

In 1996, there were 10 102 physicians in family practice residencies. Starting with 15 programs, the specialty had grown to 452 in facilities throughout the United States. Family practice residents learn not only the "high-tech" skills of 20th-century medicine, but also the "high-touch" skills integral to successful family medicine. Among the techniques used is mock hospitalization, in which residents undergo the experience of hospital admission during their orientation.

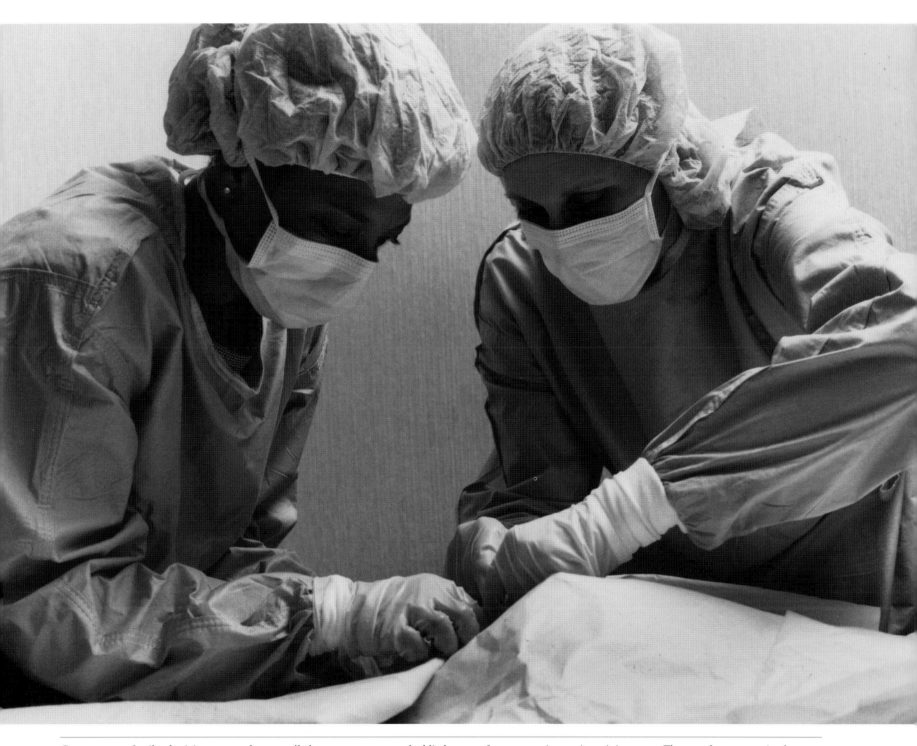

Contemporary family physicians are no longer called on to amputate crushed limbs or perform an ovariotomy in a sitting room. They are, however, trained to assist at surgery and carry out limited surgical procedures, to recognize conditions requiring referral to a surgeon, to provide pre- and postoperative management, and to give advice and emotional support to their patients in need of surgery.

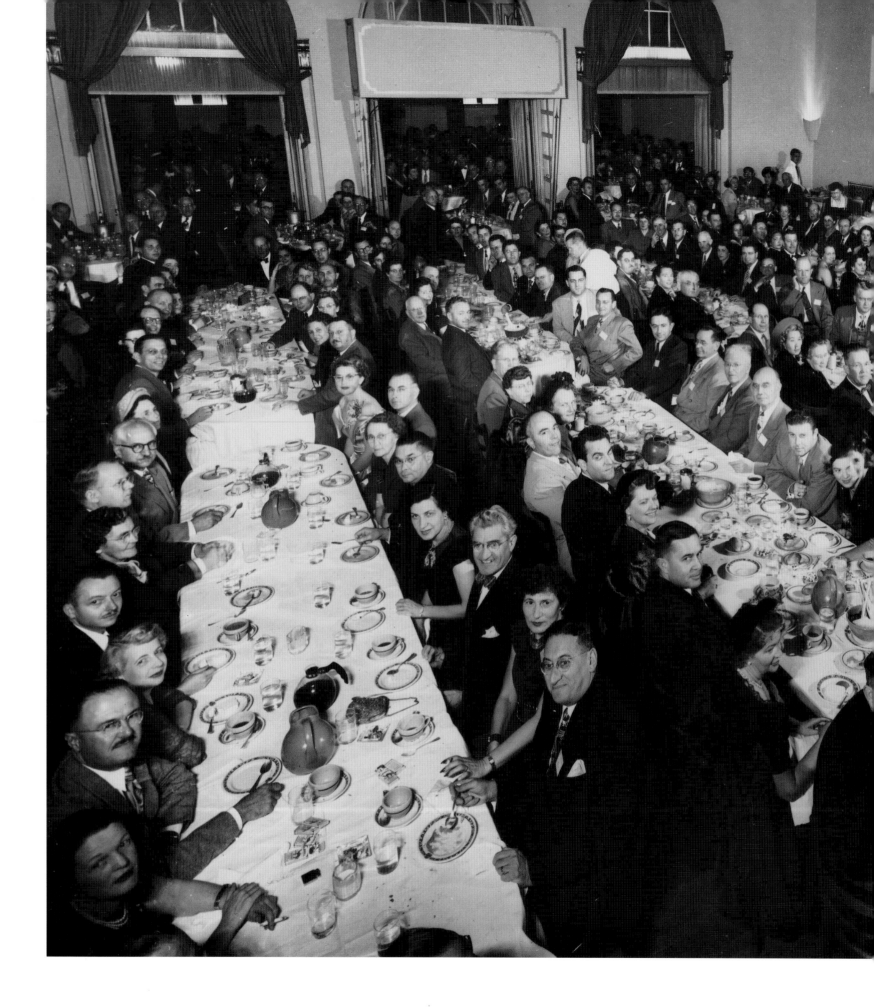

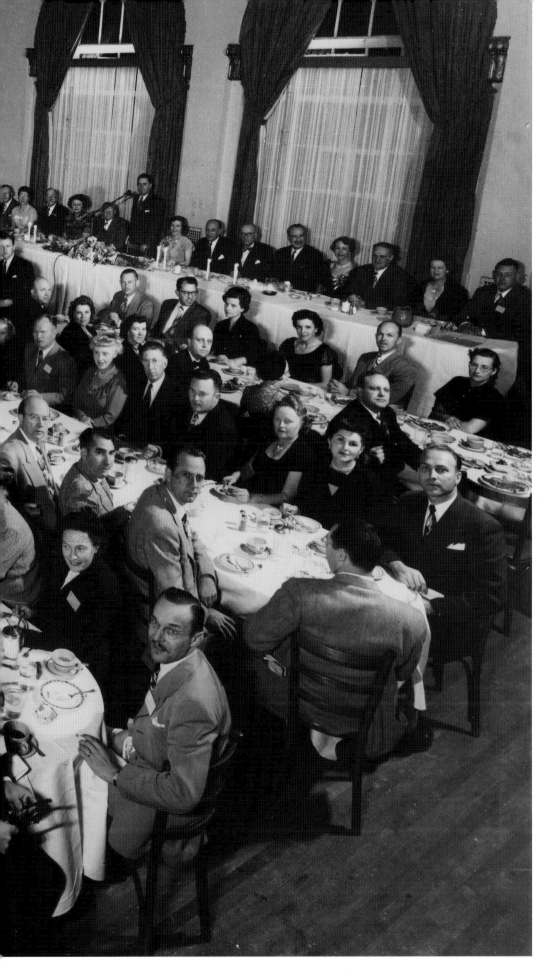

In 1950 when these physicians and their spouses took part in the Scientific Assembly of the California Academy of General Practice (now Family Physicians), American medical practice was undergoing significant post–World War II changes. For example, new drugs such as penicillin meant more patients could be cured than ever before. In addition, improved laboratory tests and sophisticated instruments contributed to the physicians' diagnostic capabilities. Finally, many of these California physicians and their colleagues throughout the country were or soon would be practicing in partnerships and groups.

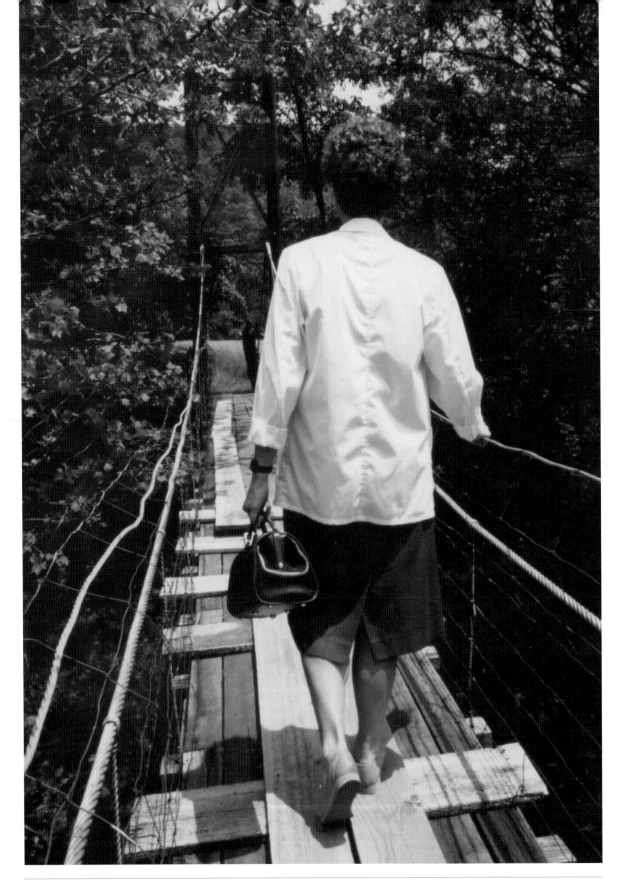

Since the first cities arose in America, there have been significant disparities in physician distribution. Early in this century, one journalist predicted the disappearance of the country doctor as early as 1923, a prediction that has not come true. Nevertheless, rural communities today use a variety of incentives—from funding a student's medical education to building hospitals—in order to lure physicians, especially family physicians, to settle in their town.

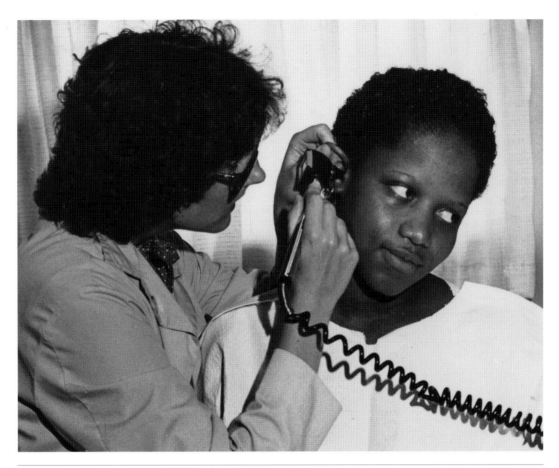

Throughout their history, family physicians have played a pivotal role in providing care to urban dwellers, especially the poor and those newly arrived in the United States. In the 1880s and 1890s, urban settlement houses were established, largely church supported and run by well-educated women. Among their services was basic health care. Today much of the medical care for America's urban poor is provided through clinics, operated by hospitals and government agencies and staffed by family and other physicians.

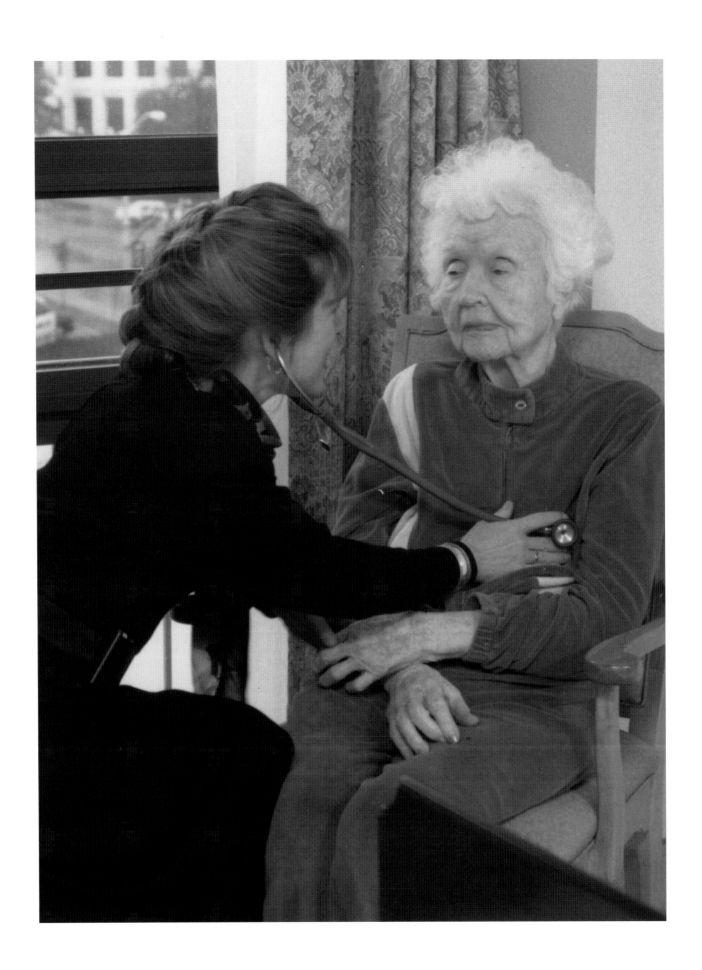

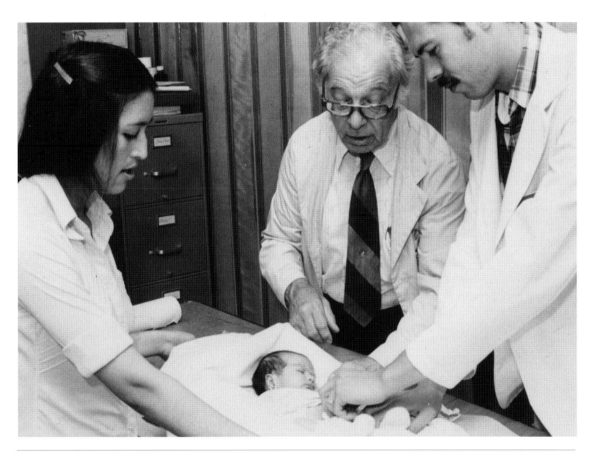

Left: One of the effects of the aging of America is the addition of the nursing facility as a practice site for increasing numbers of physicians. About 5 percent of America's elderly are being cared for in nearly 20 000 nursing facilities. It is estimated that nearly one third of Americans will need a nursing facility at some time after age 65. Because a greater variety of long-term care alternatives to nursing home care is available, most elderly who reside in nursing facilities are significantly impaired or ill and require close monitoring by their physicians.

Above: America's migrant farm workers have long had one of the highest death rates in the country. Their itinerant lifestyle poses special problems for the physicians who seek to provide continuity of care, as in this Michigan clinic for migrant workers.

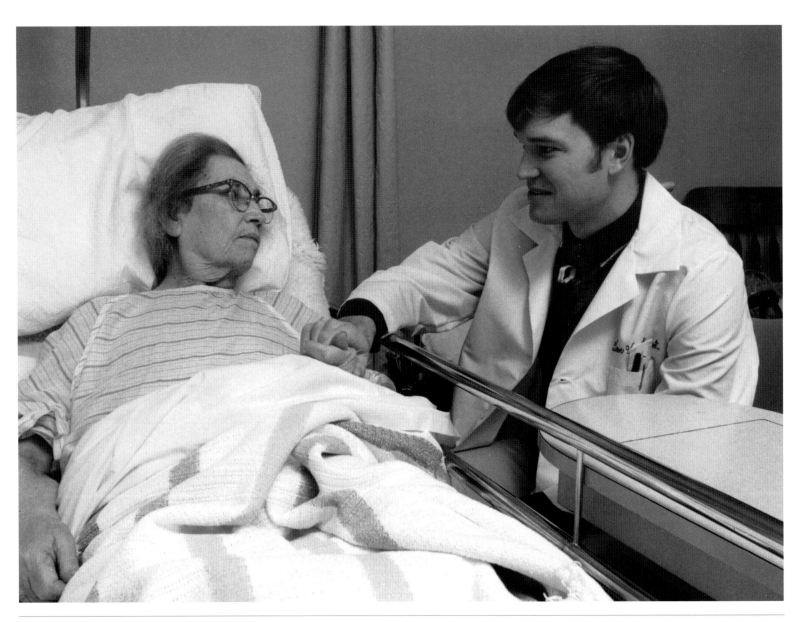

The 1980s and 1990s have seen a steady decline in the average length of a hospital stay, from 6.7 days in 1980 to 5.1 in 1995. Nevertheless, family physicians are important advocates on behalf of their hospitalized patients, who tend to be sicker on average than those hospitalized during the 1960s and 1970s.

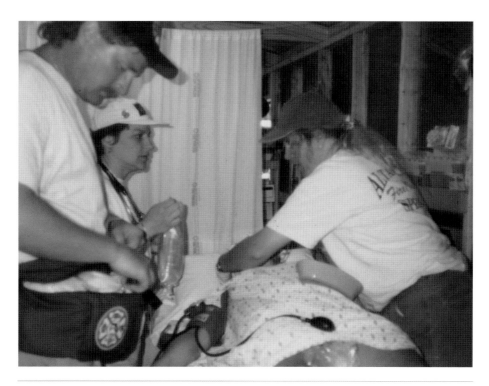

Their breadth of medical training stands family physicians in good stead as they take part in a wide range of community activities. For example, Tennessee family physician Dr. Karen Gilson, center, and paramedics Jerry Bills and Cindy Bilanki were among several thousand health care professionals who staffed medical field units during the 1996 Centennial Olympics field trials and games.

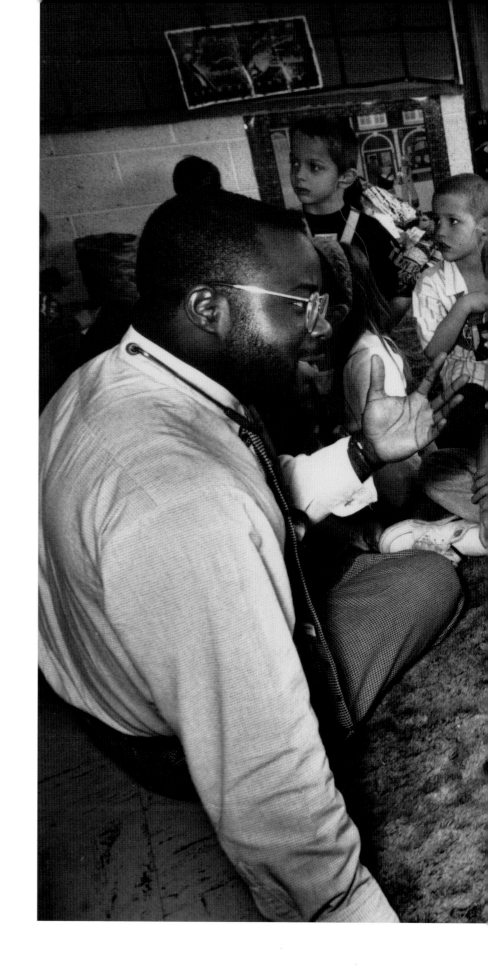

Preventive medicine, wellness education, and lifestyle concerns are important elements in medicine under managed care of the 1990s. Family physicians are often in the forefront of community efforts to bring the wellness message to even young residents. For example, the Ohio School Visit Program brings medical students into public school classrooms for an early lesson in good health.

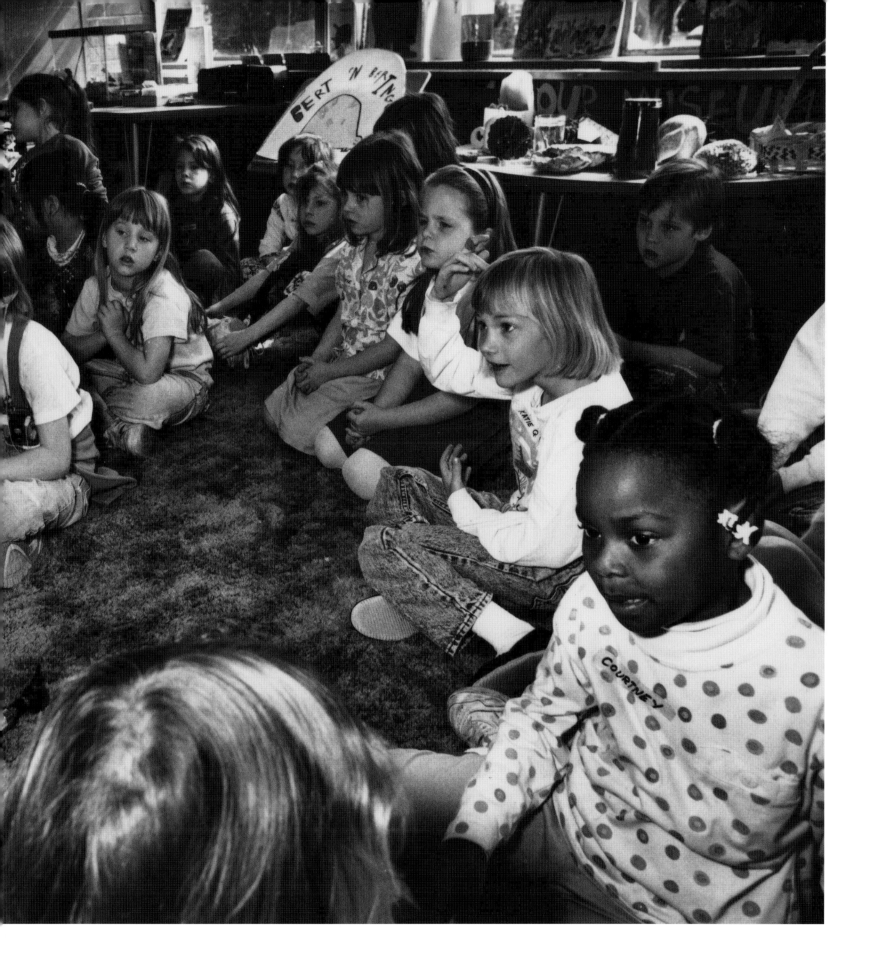

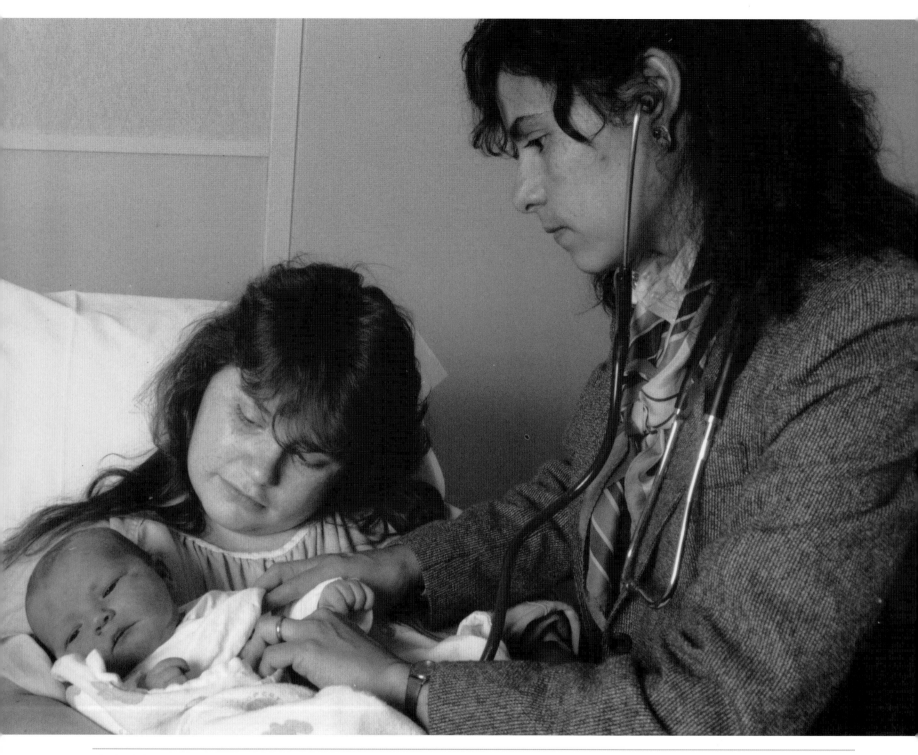

The final three decades of the 20th century marked another life milestone for the "Baby Boom" generation as its members entered their childbearing years. Many family physicians continue in the tradition of earlier general practitioners to provide total obstetrical care for these mothers as well as care for the children.

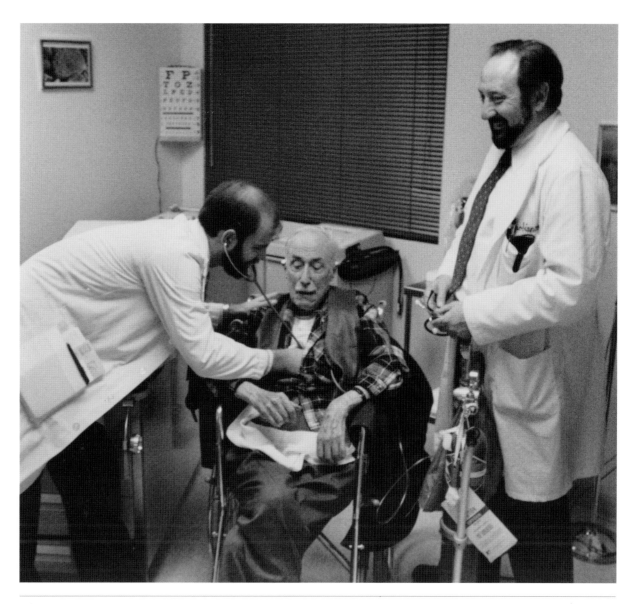

Of necessity, contemporary family physicians see an increasing number of elderly patients. In 1965 when Medicare began, 18 million Americans were 65 or over. Thirty years later, that number is 34 million and rising, as the oldest members of the "Baby Boom" generation enter their 50s. One medical trendwatcher notes that the elderly constitute 40-50 percent of physician revenues.

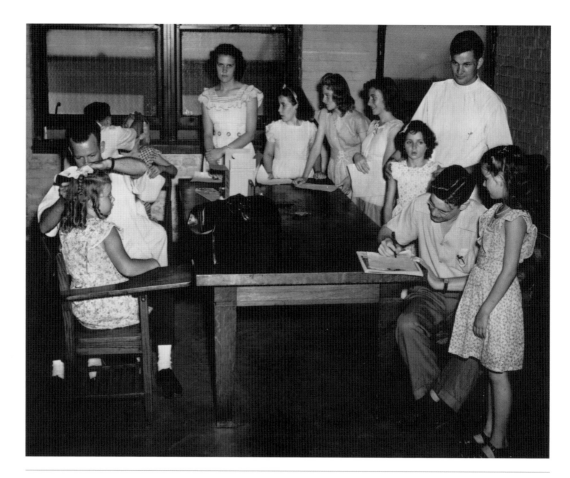

The preschool physical examination has been an important responsibility for family physicians throughout most of this century. Community clinics such as this 1950s one in Missouri provided an opportunity for physicians to see children who might otherwise be unable to afford any medical care.

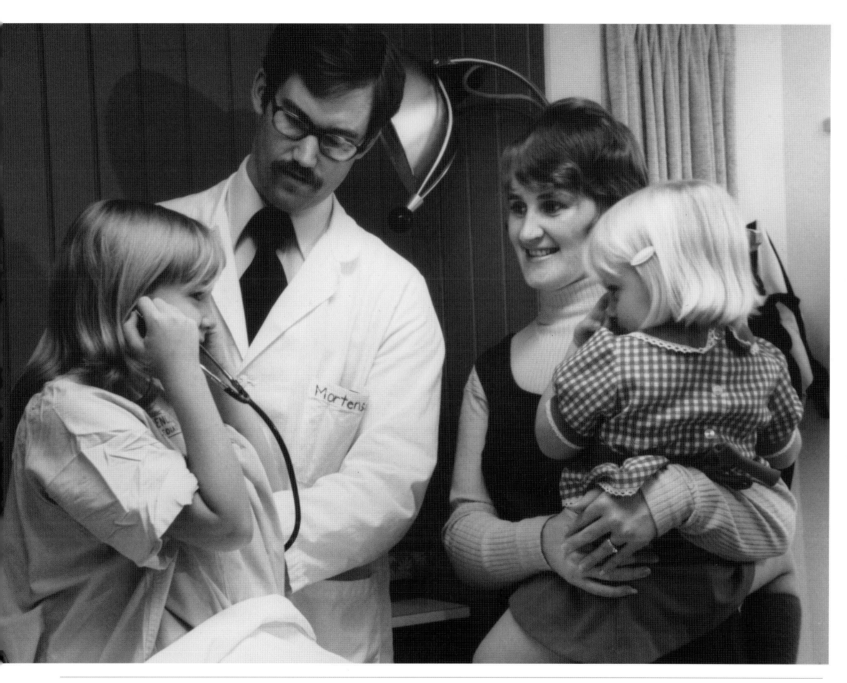

Getting ready for school still includes a visit to the doctor for many American children, to update immunizations and carry out physical examinations. Young athletes also undergo screening for authorization to take part in soccer and other sports. These visits are ideal opportunities for the family physician to provide some basic health and wellness education as well.

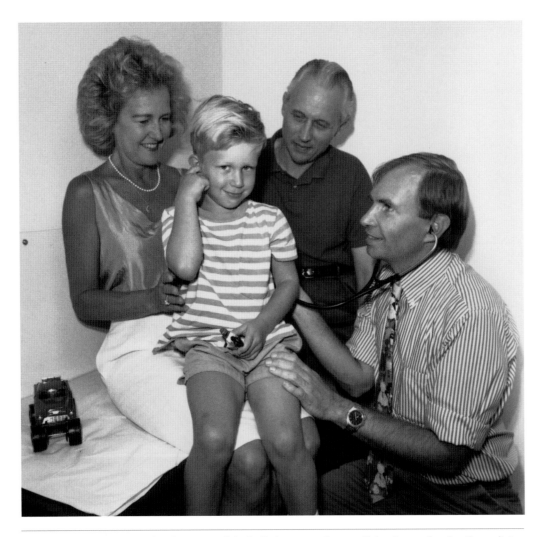

Getting to know the entire family is part of the holistic approach to medicine integral to family medicine from its earliest beginnings. Family physicians encourage families to participate in one another's care and to bring questions and concerns to the physician's attention.

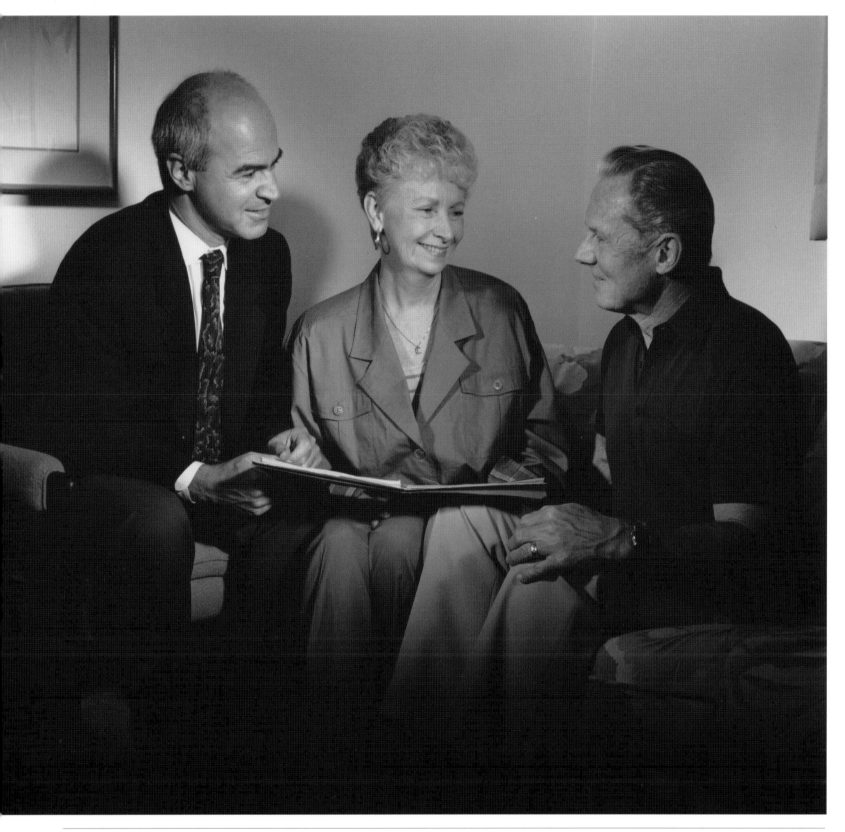

In 1980 a study involving patients in a family practice center found that there was an important link between the patients' perceptions of socioemotional aspects of the physician-patient relationship and their satisfaction with care. Specifically, patients who felt their physicians were effective communicators also believed that they were providing appropriate, effective care. Patient satisfaction was highly related to their feelings that their physicians communicated with them and cared about them as people. This has important implications for busy practitioners, not only because satisfaction relates to patient retention, but also because other studies have shown a relationship between patient satisfaction and compliance and recovery.

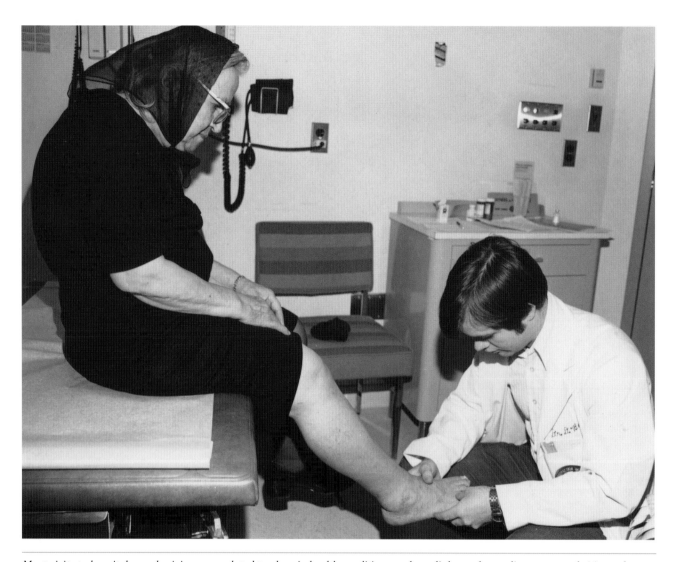

Most visits to hospitals or physicians are related to chronic health conditions such as diabetes, heart disease, or arthritis, and 80 percent of all deaths are due to these types of conditions. In particular, more than 80 percent of the older population suffer from one or more of these illnesses, with half of those age 65 or older suffering from arthritis. Family physicians are called on to monitor these conditions, educate their patients to limit disabilities and complications, and manage these conditions as patients undergo various medical therapies.

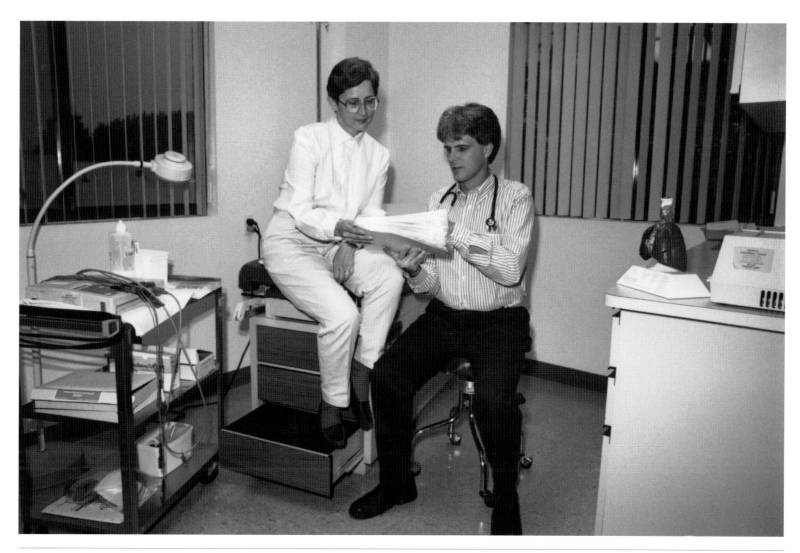

Careful patient education helps ensure compliance and an effective physician-patient collaboration, fundamental to family practice. The final two decades of the 20th century have experienced a rise in medical consumerism and a growing emphasis on personal responsibility for overall well-being, both of which are fundamental tenets of family medicine. For its part, the federal government hopes to have three out of four physicians involved in patient education by the year 2000.

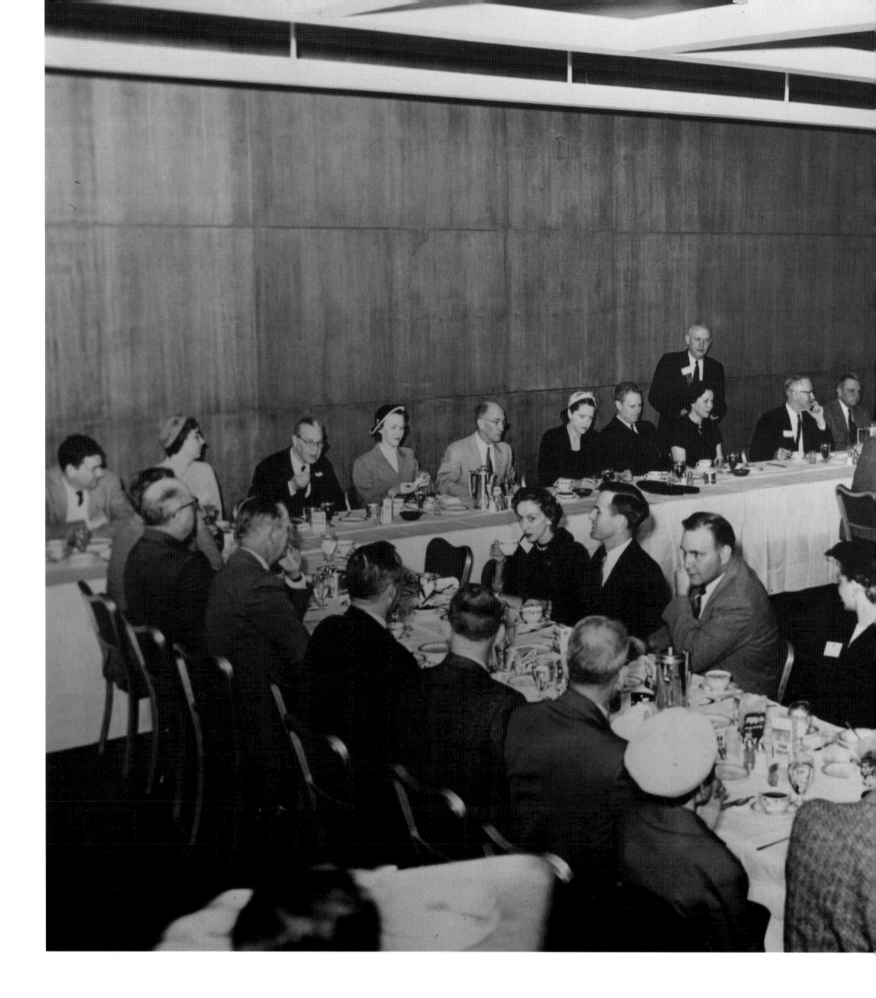

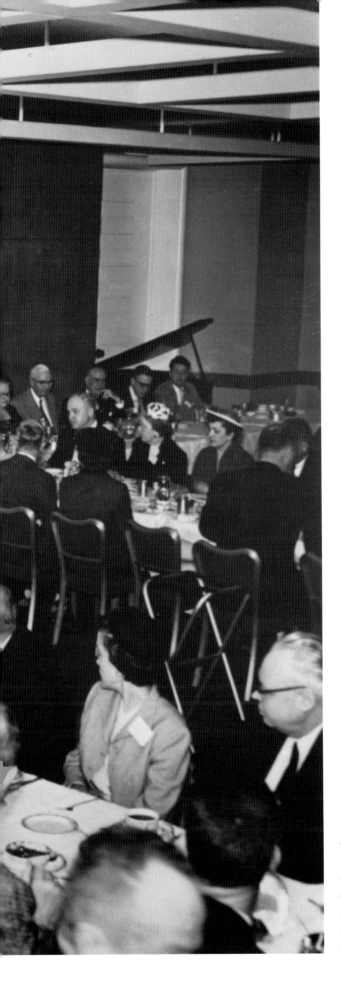

World War II brought about a significant change in the relationship among the various components of medical care—physicians, hospitals, research, government, and industry—with increasing interdependency. At the same time, power shifted somewhat as the American Medical Association became one of several medical interest groups lobbying on behalf of its members. At this 1952 Leadership Breakfast in Washington, DC, members of the Tennessee Academy of Family Physicians met with Tennessee Senator Albert Gore, Sr. (seated at right of speaker).

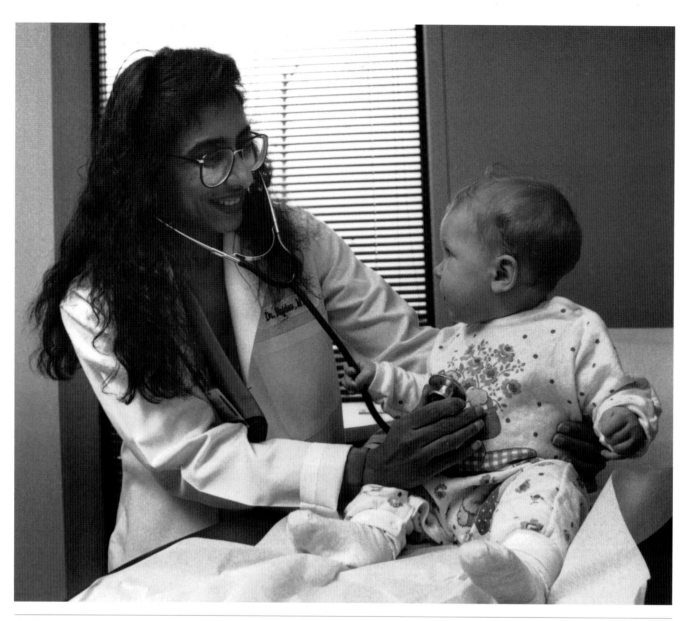

At the beginning of this century, women comprised 4 percent of all medical graduates. With numerous up-and-down fluctuations, by 1990 over 35 percent of medical graduates were women. Their impact was particularly felt in the primary care specialties: 54 percent of pediatric residents, 47 percent of ob-gyn residents, 35 percent of family practice residents, and 29 percent of internal medicine residents were women in 1990.

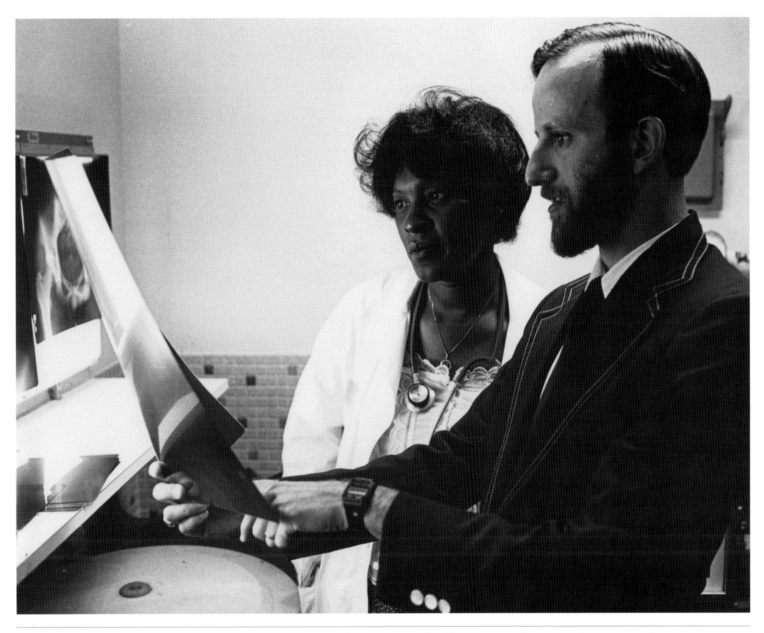

The solo practitioner is becoming increasingly rare and even those who maintain a solo office rarely care for their patients entirely alone. Managed care, by putting the family physician in the role of coordinator of a patient's care, has assured that this physician most often participates in team care with other health care professionals.

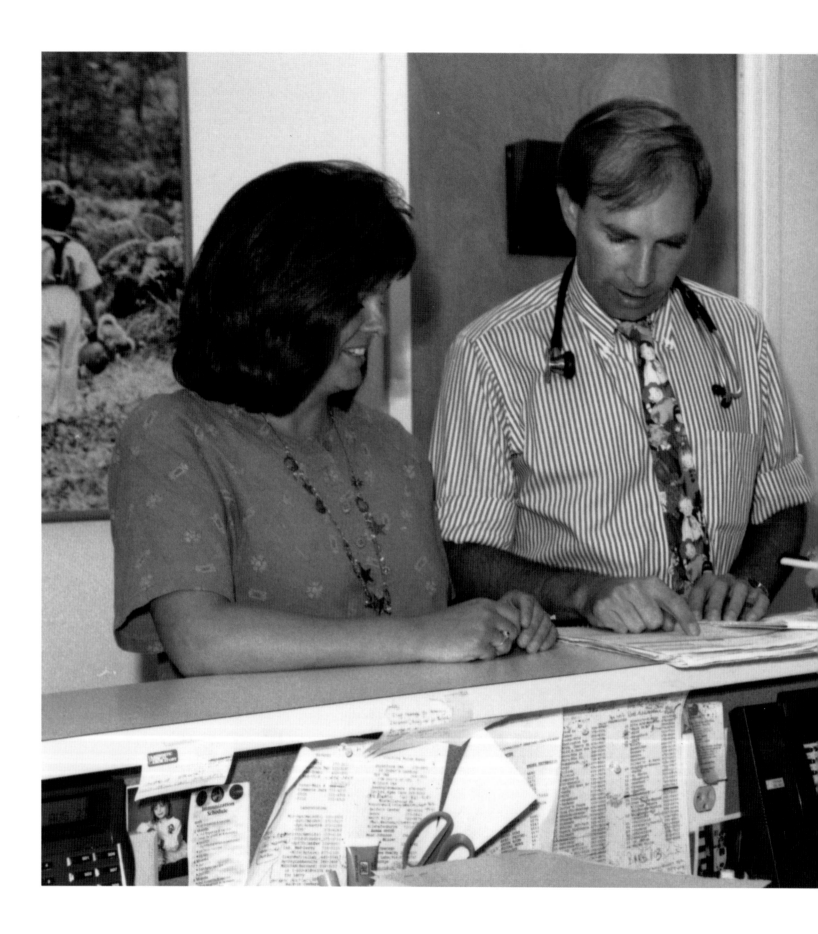

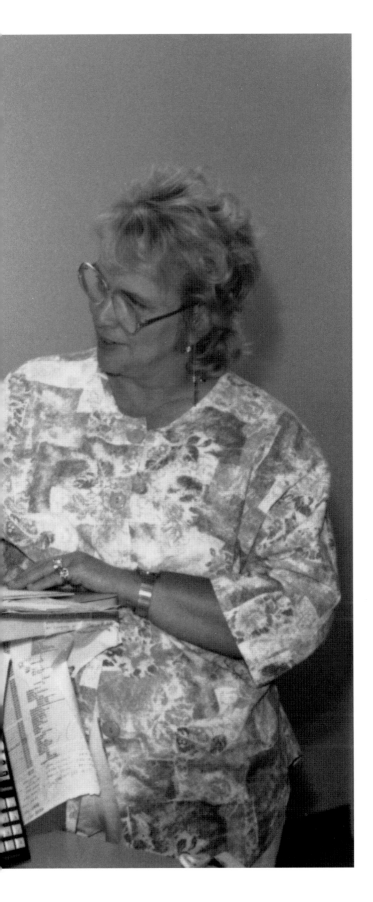

While the predecessor to today's family physician may have ridden the prairies alone or managed an office practice singlehandedly, patients visiting their physician's office now are likely to find nurse practitioners, nurse assistants, laboratory technicians, medical records specialists, business managers, office managers, insurance claims specialists, and receptionists. Medical offices, including those of family physicians, are major employers, and many medical support professions are expected to be growth employment areas into the next century.

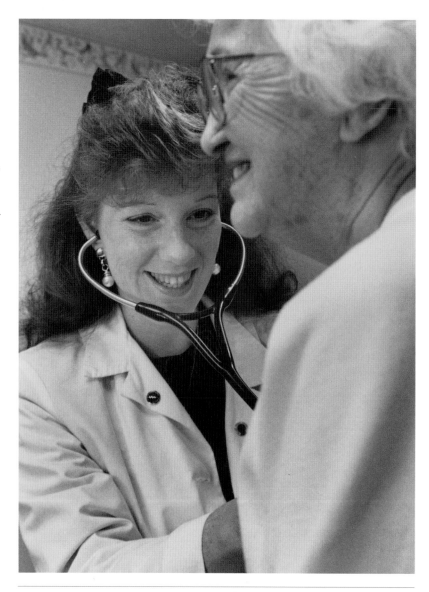

Above and right: Despite repeated predictions for the disappearance of the family physician, these doctors continue to provide a significant level of health care for many Americans. With the critical role these physicians play in the managed care system, most trendwatchers predict even greater opportunities for family physicians. From earliest times on North American shores to today, the challenges of caring for patients of all ages and with a multitude of health concerns are significant. But so have been the opportunities to become an important figure in the lives of many.

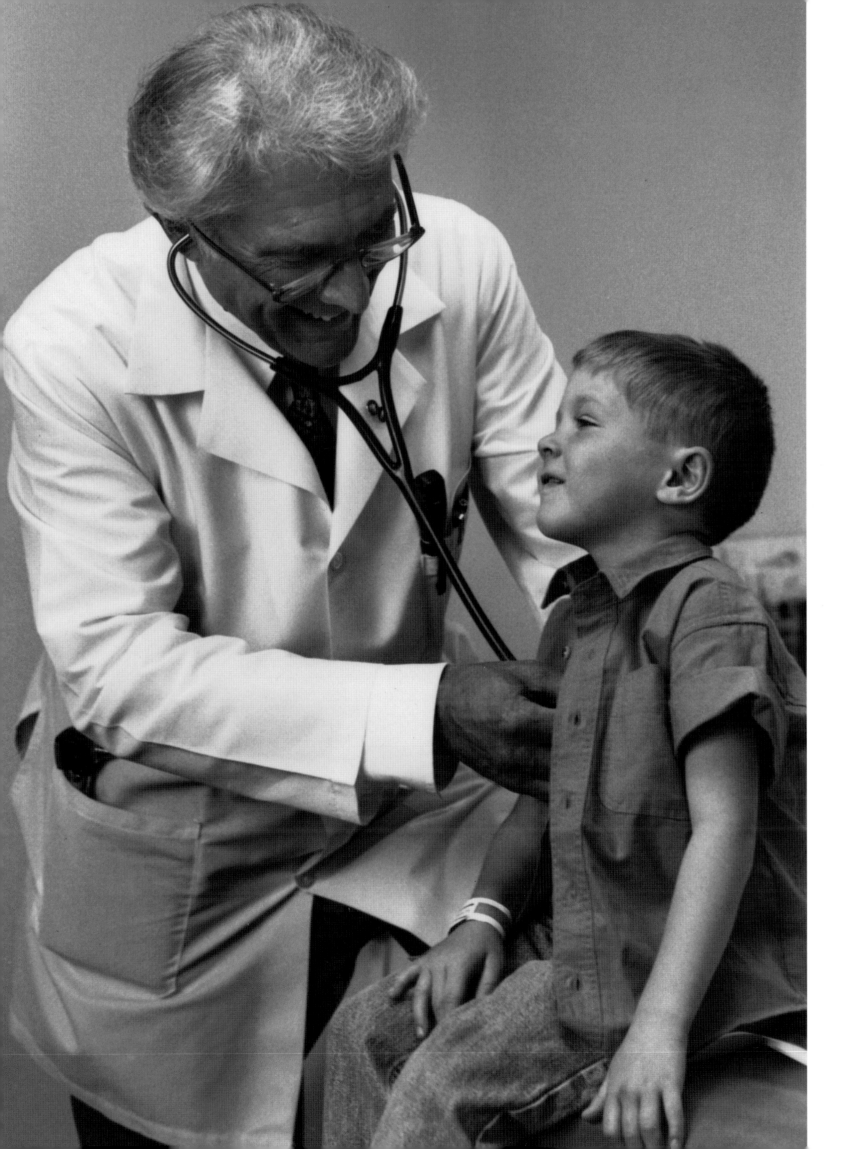

Related Readings

Ackerknecht EH. *A Short History of Medicine.* Rev. ed. New York, NY: Ronald Press; 1982.

Apple RD, ed. *Women, Health and Medicine in America: A Historical Handbook.* New York, NY: Rutgers University Press; 1990.

Bettman OC. *A Pictorial History of Medicine.* Springfield, Ill: Charles C. Thomas; 1956.

Bordley J III, Harvey AM. *Two Centuries of American Medicine: 1776-1976.* Philadelphia, Penn: WB Saunders; 1976.

Cassedy JH. *Medicine in America: A Short History.* Baltimore, Md: The Johns Hopkins University Press; 1991.

Clarke H. *The Apothecary in Eighteenth-Century Williamsburg.* Williamsburg, Va: Colonial Williamsburg; 1965.

Corcoran AC. *A Mirror Up to Medicine.* New York, NY: JB Lippincott Co; 1961.

Davis AB. *Medicine and Its Technology.* Westport, Conn: Greenwood Press; 1981.

Duffy J. *Epidemics in Colonial America.* Baton Rouge, La: Louisiana State University Press; 1953.

Duffy J. *From Humors to Medical Science.* 2nd ed. Urbana, Ill: University of Illinois Press; 1993.

Duncan LC. *Medical Men in the American Revolution, 1775-1783.* Reprint of 1931 ed. Barracks, Penn: Augustus Kelley Publishers; 1970.

Flexner JT. *Doctors on Horseback: Pioneers of American Medicine.* Reprint of 1957 ed. New York, NY: Dover Publications; 1969.

Gevitz N. *The D.O.s: Osteopathic Medicine in America.* Baltimore, Md: Johns Hopkins University Press; 1982.

Gevitz N, ed. *Unorthodox Medicine in America.* Baltimore, Md: Johns Hopkins University Press; 1988.

Haagensen CD, Lloyd WE. *A Hundred Years of Medicine.* New York, NY: Sheridan; 1943.

Haggard HW. *Devils, Drugs, and Doctors: The Story of the Science of Healing from Medicine-Man to Doctor.* New York, NY: Blue Ribbon Books; 1929.

Haller JS Jr. *American Medicine in Transition, 1840-1910.* Urbana, Ill: University of Illinois Press; 1981.

Kalman B. *Early Health and Medicine.* New York, NY: Crabtree Publishing; 1983.

Karolevitz RF. *Doctors of the Old West.* New York, NY: Bonanza Books; 1967.

Kett JE. *The Formation of the American Medical Profession: The Role of Institutions, 1780-1960.* New Haven, Conn: Yale University Press; 1968.

King LS. *The Medical World of the 18th Century.* Chicago, Ill: University of Chicago Press; 1958.

Ludmerer K. *Learning to Heal: The Development of American Medical Education.* Baltimore, Md: Johns Hopkins University Press; 1996.

Lyons AS, Petrucelli J II. *Medicine: An Illustrated History.* New York, NY: Abradale Press, Harry N. Abrams; 1987.

Marks G, Beatty W. *The Story of Medicine in America.* New York, NY: Scribners; 1973.

Marti–Ibanez F. *The Epic of Medicine.* New York: Clarkson Potter; 1962.

Morais HM. *The History of the Afro-American in Medicine.* Rev. ed. New York, NY: Publishers Agency; 1976.

Murphy L. *Enter the Physician: The Transformation of Domestic Medicine, 1760-1860.* Tuscaloosa, Ala: University of Alabama Press; 1991.

Novotny A, Smith C, eds. *Images of Healing: A Portfolio of American Medical & Pharmaceutical Practice in the 18th, 19th, & Early 20th Centuries.* New York, NY: Macmillan; 1980.

Osler W. *The Evolution of Modern Medicine.* New Haven, Conn: Yale University Press; 1921.

Pusey WA. *A Doctor in the 1870s and 1880s.* Springfield, Ill: Charles C. Thomas; 1932.

Rosenberg CE. *The Care of Strangers: The Rise of America's Hospital System.* New York, NY: Basic Books; 1987.

Rosenberg L. *The Story of Modern Medicine.* New York, NY: WW Norton; 1966.

Rothstein WG. *American Physicians in the Nineteenth Century: From Sects to Science.* Baltimore, Md: Johns Hopkins University Press; 1992.

Smolan R, Moffitt P. *Medicine's Great Journey.* Boston, Mass: Little Brown & Company; 1992.

Stoeckle J. *Plain Pictures of Plain Doctoring: Vernacular Expression in New Deal Medicine and Photography.* Cambridge, Mass: MIT Press; 1990.

Photo Credits

A.T. Still Memorial Library, Kirksville College of Osteopathic Medicine, Kirksville, Missouri–47, 62–63, 110

California Academy of Family Physicians, San Francisco, California–98–99

Colorado Historical Society, Denver, Colorado–36–37, 40

The Connecticut Historical Society, Hartford, Connecticut–16

Michael J. Connolly, MD, Stratford, Connecticut. Photographer: Debranne Cingari–115

Corbis-Bettmann, New York, New York–79 right

The Denver Public Library, Western History Department, Denver, Colorado–51, 73

Harvard Medical Library in the Francis A. Countway Library of Medicine, Boston, Massachusetts–89

Bob Hitchcock, Altamonte Springs Fire Department, Altamonte Springs, Florida–105

Illinois State Historical Library, Springfield, Illinois–38

Kansas State Historical Society, Topeka, Kansas–25, 48–49

Library of Congress, Washington, DC–23, 27, 28, 31, 33, 35, 57

Library of Congress, Washington, DC. Probable photographer: W.H. Willard Jones–Cover, 67

Library of Congress, Washington, DC. Photographer: Arthur Rothstein–65, 85

R. Scott Prewitt, MD, Stratford, Connecticut. Photographer: Debranne Cingari–93, 112, 121

St. Vincent's Medical Center, Bridgeport, Connecticut–74, 75, 76–77

St. Vincent's Medical Center, Bridgeport, Connecticut. Photographer: Debranne Cingari–84

St. Vincent's Medical Center, Bridgeport, Connecticut. Photographer: Peter Tepper–92

Smithsonian Institution, NMAH/Medical Sciences, Washington, DC–46 (Photo no. 63915), 55 (Photo no. 79-5036), 56 (Photo no. 78-10551)

State Historical Society of North Dakota, Bismarck, North Dakota–42 bottom

State Historical Society of Wisconsin, Madison, Wisconsin–41

Tennessee Academy of Family Physicians, Brentwood, Tennessee–116–117

University of Nebraska Medical Center, Omaha, Nebraska–61

University of North Texas Health Science Center, Fort Worth, Texas–102

University of Oklahoma Library, Western History Collections, Norman, Oklahoma–68, 70, 78–79 left, 81, 82

Utah State Historical Society, Salt Lake City, Utah. All rights reserved. Used by permission.–42 top, 59, 60 bottom

West Virginia School of Osteopathic Medicine, Lewisburg, West Virginia–100

W.H. Over State Museum, Vermillion, South Dakota–43